THE WHOLE BODY RESTART
FOR HEALTHY AGING

THE 14-DAY PROVEN DIET PLAN TO LOSE WEIGHT,
RESET METABOLISM, AND IMPROVE PHYSICAL &
MENTAL HEALTH AT MIDLIFE... AND BEYOND

PAGE WEST

CONTENTS

JUST FOR YOU

A FREE GIFT TO OUR READERS

07 amazing recipes to be warm and healthy and enjoy the cold days among family and friends!

WARM & HEALTHY WINTER WITH DELICIOUS SOUPS!

Download here:

PAGEWESTPUBLISHING.COM/GIFT

INTRODUCTION

"If we could give every individual the right amount of nourishment and exercise, not too little and not too much, we would have found the safest way to health."

— HIPPOCRATES

Are you feeling like you don't have the energy for your busy life? Maybe you're tired, and you're pretty sure all that excess weight has something to do with it! You'd love to take it off, but somehow it seems harder now that you're older.

You may have been one of the "lucky" ones who never seemed to gain weight in your twenties and thirties, but you're no longer feeling so lucky! Or maybe you've been overweight for a long time, but it has never bothered you. Either way, you're not alone. Adult obesity rates are highest between the ages of 45 and 54.[1]

Why is midlife so conducive to extra weight? There are a number of reasons why you might have only recently seen the pounds creeping up on you. The human body's metabolism tends to slow down with age, for one thing. Lifestyle factors may be influencing weight as well: anything from settling down with a long-term partner or (conversely) divorcing, parenthood, dealing with elderly parents... the list goes on.

The good news is that you don't have to keep all these midlife pounds! Getting rid of them may be a little trickier than it was a decade or two ago, but that doesn't make it impossible. You may need a different strategy, and that's where this book comes in.

Losing weight when you're older requires a few more strategies, some of which are really not about the weight at all but being able to handle the stress that comes with modern life for those past the age of forty. That's why you'll find chapters about dancing, stretching, and mindfulness. Are they directly related to weight loss? Not as much as the chapters on detoxifying and clean eating—but they can keep you more relaxed, so you're not tempted to go off the meal plan.

By implementing the easy-to-use practical tips in this book, not only will you get a jump start on losing weight, but you'll understand the tools you need to keep it off. So many people lose weight on a diet, only to find that the weight comes back on when they go "off" the diet. In fact, that may have happened to you as well!

The reason is that you don't learn the techniques that help you keep from eating when you get stressed out, or the diet doesn't show you how to eat for the rest of your life. That's where diets fail, but the Whole Body Jumpstart can show you how to continue eating and moving the right way for the rest of your life, so the pounds don't come back on.

The meal plans and recipes cover detoxifying smoothies to address your hunger and nutritional needs in the morning. Then you get lunch, dinner, and a snack as well. It's enough food to keep you satisfied and not feeling deprived, but with enough nutritional content that you're returning your body back to physical health. With all of the conflicting messages in the media and habits that you've built up over time, you may no longer be in touch with the kind of food that's satisfying and good for you. But don't worry, we include shopping lists so you can ensure that you've got all the ingredients you need for the right food on your meal plan.

At this point, you might be wondering why you should dive into this book. How do I, the author, know enough to make good on my promise of physical and mental health? I personally understand the frustrations that people feel when in middle age when the number on the scale keeps creeping up…and up…and up. Even when they're on a diet or eating special food.

After years of personal frustration, I found a new love for wellness and have discovered how much doing mindful exercises and focusing on whole foods can get that scale to budge. And, more importantly, enjoying a healthy life.

I want to help many more people find joy and health in their middle years. Therefore, I've written a book to reach as many people as I can, with an easy-to-follow plan that will help them find success by changing their lifestyle and mindset for good.

What are you waiting for? Let's get started so you can begin to drop the weight and get healthy!

---

1. https://www.wihealthatlas.org/obesity/age

HOW AGING MAKES WEIGHT GAIN WORSE

"It's going to be a journey. It's not a sprint to get in shape."

— KERRI WALSH JENNINGS

The fact is that human bodies change as they age. Sometimes people get plastic surgery, which may affect the visible changes, but not all changes can be fixed with surgery. Some age-related alterations happen at the cellular level, or to organs and systems inside the body.

Whether or not plastic surgery is your reality, you still need to understand what's going on with your body in order to maintain both physical and mental health. Menopause is a very specific set of changes, so in this chapter, you'll discover some age-related issues that are just for women.

Outward changes: body shape, weight, and fat distribution

Your body essentially comprises fat, water, lean tissue such as muscles and organs, and bones. After age 30, people tend to lose lean tissue, which means a loss of muscle mass and the loss of cells in your organs such as kidneys and lungs. But we tend to gain fat, whereas older people can have as much as a third more fat compared to when they were younger.[1]

Not only that, but many of us become shorter, largely due to age-related differences in joints, muscles, and bones. It's possible to lose one to three inches in height as you get older. Fortunately, that doesn't have to happen, if you're eating right and treating bone loss.

But the result of having less muscle mass and stiff joints, plus more fat distributed differently, can make keeping your balance harder. That's why so many elderly people fall so often—they're off-balance, which is at least partly due to these body shape changes.

For women especially, midlife can change their body shape simply by redistributing excess fat. In their childbearing years, women often carry more weight on their hips and thighs. But by perimenopause—the years right before menopause—weight often shifts to the tummy. You might go from a pear shape, where excess fat is less dangerous to your health, to an apple shape.

You can see why it's important to take the weight off and maintain that weight loss as you grow older. You are fighting the effects of aging to a certain degree, but losing weight can help you stay healthier and be less prone to falls and other injuries.

Inward changes

All human bodies have additional age-related changes. The good news is that you can combat many of these changes with good physical and mental health. Being in a good position healthwise can also lessen the effects of some of these changes. Also, most of the changes that we discuss below occur throughout your lifetime, so you might not be experiencing them right now in midlife. Or if you are, the alterations are small.

- Cells

If you've ever had an older car, you know it takes more TLC to maintain it and keep it going. That goes for cells too—they don't operate as well when they're older.

Cells can die as well. Sometimes they're programmed to do so, and sometimes it happens when they're damaged, for example by too much radiation from the sun. They can also be damaged by their own activities, such as generating free radicals when they make energy.

- Organs

Cells make up all the body's organs, so an organ's health depends on the health of the cells. Cells in the organs die and aren't always replaced, so the number of cells decreases as you age. When there aren't enough healthy cells, the organ stops working.

The organs tend to peak functionally around age 30 and decline gradually afterward. Fortunately, there's enough functional reserve in them so that there are enough cells to keep working into old age. Generally, when the organs stop working it's due to disorders or diseases rather than the normal process of aging.

- Skin

As you age, skin becomes drier, thinner, less elastic, and often finely wrinkled. Exposure to the sun ages skin much faster. Both collagen, which is a tough, fibrous material, and elastin, which makes the skin more flexible, tend to decrease as you grow older, which makes skin tearing more likely.

Nerve endings under the skin decrease over time as well, which makes people less sensitive to pain, pressure, and extreme temperatures. That makes injuries more likely. As the number of sweat glands and blood vessels decreases below the skin (and elsewhere), blood flow to the skin decreases as well. With less blood flow, people have a harder time cooling off when they get overheated so heat stroke and heat exhaustion become more likely too.

The body produces less of the skin pigment melanin as it ages, so the skin has less protection against the sun's damaging ultraviolet rays. At the same time, it's harder to make vitamin D from sunlight.

- Immune system

Like many of the other processes in the body, your immune system works more slowly as you age. Because of this, cancer is more common in older people, and vaccines are less effective—though vaccines are still your best protection against certain viruses like shingles, some forms of pneumonia, and the flu. Infections from the flu or pneumonia (or others) may be more severe in older people, resulting in death.

Yet there's a silver lining to this cloud: people who suffer from immune disorders, including allergies, suffer less as the immune system slows down.

- Brain and nervous system

Although neurons (brain cells) can die, that doesn't necessarily mean that you have an overall loss of brain cells.

Neurons can regenerate. New connections are often made between existing cells, plus the brain has extra cells to protect against losing too many.

Even so, as blood flow decreases with age and neurons lose some of their receptors, your brain won't function quite as fast as it did when you were younger. But don't worry, older people are still able to function! They just tend to be slower than their younger counterparts.

After about age 60, the spine starts losing nerve cells (gradually). Nerves often conduct their messaging and signaling more slowly as well, so older people may have decreased sensation and strength.

- Muscles

While muscle mass does decrease, older people can still remain athletic and are able to "go hard," though to a lesser degree compared to when they were younger. Staying physically active means you'll likely be active longer—being sedentary can lead to less mobility as you grow older.

When you're older, being inactive takes a bigger toll than it did when you were younger. It's harder to come back from a period of no physical activity. (So the obvious solution is not to stop!) You lose muscle mass much more quickly, so it's key to do resistance training as you grow older in addition to the cardiovascular activity that helps your heart.

- Bones and joints

Your bones are less dense as you get older, which can mean they're weaker and more easily broken. As women go through menopause, their bones get more brittle due to the loss of estrogen, which normally prevents bone tissue from breaking down too easily.

The body can't absorb as much calcium and vitamin D as you grow older, which is why bones get weaker. If the top of your spine gets too weak, your head can tip forward. This compresses the throat, which can make you more likely to choke.

Also, the lining around your joints (cartilage) gets thinner, which can make moving those joints more painful. Ligaments and tendons become less elastic, so you're less flexible and more likely to tear these tissues.

- Heart

With age, your heart and blood vessels get stiffer. Since the heart fills with blood more slowly and the arteries are slower to expand, many people find their blood pressure increases. Even so, your heart still keeps functioning. But keeping it healthy (especially with exercise) can help you improve your performance as you grow older.

- Lungs

Muscles weaken as people age, and there are fewer air sacs and capillaries. These conditions lead to less oxygen being absorbed from each breath, and (like your heart and arteries) your lungs are less elastic. Even if you have no lung disorders or smoking history, exercise or breathing at high altitudes could be harder.

It's also harder to resist infections because coughs tend to weaken with age, and it's harder for the lungs to sweep out debris.

- Kidneys and urinary tract

Similar to some of the other systems we've discussed, the kidneys and urinary tract do change with age but usually still function. There are fewer cells in the kidneys and less blood flow, and they may not filter out toxins, which often leads to dehydration.

Older people often have bladder problems since this organ can be affected by age in various ways. It becomes smaller, so people may need to pee more often. It can become overactive or stop emptying as well, so there's some urine left even after you're "done." The muscle that controls the movement out of the body gets weaker, so it's harder to postpone urination.

In men, the prostate gland can become enlarged and prevent the bladder from working correctly. That could mean going more often, dribbling at the end, and taking longer to start.

- Digestive system

This system tends to be less affected by aging. Although the esophagus muscles are a bit less forceful and food empties out of the stomach more slowly (so you don't eat as much food as you used to), these changes tend to be small and often not even noticeable. Because the large intestine moves material through more slowly, seniors may find that constipation becomes an issue.

- Endocrine system

This system in the body controls many of the hormones that are important for health. Growth hormone production typically decreases, so there's less muscle mass. The hormone that controls salt retention doesn't work as well, so you might be dehydrated more often. The production of insulin is less effective (even if you're not diabetic), so your blood sugar may remain higher after a large meal and takes longer to drop back down into the normal range.

- Eyes

There are a variety of changes in the eye as you get older, which make it harder to focus on things that are near to you (which usually means you need reading glasses) as well as making it harder to see in dim light. Because the eye's lens gets yellower with age, your color perception could change.

The pupils react to changes in light more slowly, so you may need a longer adjustment time when entering a dark or very bright room. Glare is a problem for many older people as well. Your eyes may be drier, and you may see more specks or floaters, which fortunately don't interfere with your vision.

- Ears

Listening to loud music can damage your hearing, but there are age-related changes as well. It can be harder to hear higher-pitched sounds, and it might seem like everyone is mumbling all the time. Background noise can make listening to people harder too. And bonus: you might get more hair growing out of your ears!

- Mouth and nose

As you might have guessed by now, your taste and smell receptors decrease with age, so it's harder to taste things.

Less saliva production leads to dry mouth, which can also cause food to taste bland (or more bitter).

Be careful with your teeth and gums as you age. You lose gum tissue, which makes it easier for bacteria to get in at the gum line and cause infection. Keep up your brushing and flossing so you don't have to worry about losing teeth.

You may find your nose getting bigger and lengthening, while the tip droops. Similar to your ears, you might get more hair growing in your nose and on your upper lip and chin.

- Reproductive organs

The changes in hormones as we age can have some, well, interesting effects. In women, the ovaries and uterus shrink, and the vaginal lining becomes drier. Without proper lubrication, sex can be painful. But with preparation, older women still enjoy sex, especially since pregnancy is off the table!

Men don't experience the same sudden drop in sex hormones as women, but testosterone does decrease over time. The results may be lower sperm production, lower sex drive, and fewer erections, and the erections may be less rigid.

The ten major culprits of weight gain

Although many people believe that weight gain is simply due to a lack of "willpower," that's generally not true. One of the things people don't think about (especially when they're talking about lack of willpower) is that the modern world is very different from the world that human beings spent their first 50,000 years in.

When our ancestors were in the African savannah, there were no grocery stores and prepackaged food. They had to hunt or gather it; food wasn't readily available. Because there was no guarantee of when a human might eat next, the body stored food as fat that could be burned when there was a prolonged period of no food.

People grew to like food that tasted fatty, salty, or sweet because these foods were more likely to be calorie dense, where a little bit of the food provides a lot of energy. That's great when you don't know where your next meal is coming from. But not so great when there's equipment right in your very home that allows you to keep food cold (or hot) any time of day, free from bacteria and spoilage.

Our bodies today are still built on this model—to hold onto calories because the body never knows when it might need them. A liking for fatty, salty, and sweet foods that pack a lot of calories in a small package. The problem is that this model doesn't work well in the 21st century.

Here are ten reasons that people gain weight and become obese—and none of them are related to willpower.

1. Genetics

While children who are overweight tend to have overweight parents, the fact that there is a genetic component to obesity doesn't mean you're doomed if you have obesity in your family.[2] You may be genetically predisposed, but it doesn't have to be your destiny if you take care of yourself... starting with the whole body start!

2. Insulin

This hormone is critical for energy management, especially when telling cells to store fat. Remember, our bodies think we don't know when our next meal is coming! Unfortunately, the typical American diet leads to *insulin resistance*, which keeps energy stored in the fat cells instead of making it available for the body to use.

A great way to reduce insulin response is to eat more fiber and fewer refined or simple carbs—which you'll find in the recipes and meal plans later in the book.

3. Leptin resistance

Like insulin, leptin is a hormone linked to obesity. Unlike insulin, it's produced in your fat cells, and the heavier you are, the more of it you have in your blood.

When it's working properly, generally in people who are at a good weight, it tells the brain how much fat stores there are. But in overweight people, it doesn't send the right signals. This is known as leptin resistance.

4. Food addiction

These fatty, salty, and sweet foods tap into the same rewards system in the brain as addictive drugs such as cocaine and heroin do. For some people, it's easy to get addicted when they're already susceptible (again, genetics plays a role in addiction).

Just like a drug addict or an alcoholic, you can lose control and be driven by your brain's biochemistry and not the smart decisions you know you should be making.

5. Sugar

Too much sugar added to your food alters your biochemistry and affects your hormones. The sugar that's added to food tends to have too much fructose. This fructose is implicated in higher insulin levels and more insulin resistance, which leads to weight gain.

When you eat fructose in the form of whole fruit, you're getting the minerals and vitamins in the fruit plus all the fiber in the fruit, which slows down the sugar intake. But added sugar has no benefit and is unnecessary.

6. Engineered food

We Americans tend to eat a lot of heavily processed food, which is designed to stay on the shelf for a while (shelf stable), be relatively cheap to buy, and be so tasty that you'll keep buying them.

You may recall that earlier in this section we discussed how potent foods that are fatty, salty, and sweet are for human beings. Guess which tastes most of our engineered food is designed to hit! You know it—fatty, salty, sweet, and often more than one of those at a time.

7. Food availability

When food is not easily available, it's a lot easier to eat the right amount, plus you may be able to burn off calories simply by obtaining your food—hunting or gathering it. But here in the 21st century, even if your pantry or refrigerator doesn't have much in it, you can get some food very quickly.

And even more unfortunately, junk food is often cheaper than good nutritious food. People who live in "food deserts" and don't have ready access to supermarkets with a variety of good food end up eating too much junk food because that's what's available to them.

8. Aggressive marketing

There's no such thing as Big Vegetable, constantly on the airwaves and on your social media urging you to eat more nutritious greens. Junk and engineered food companies, on the other hand, are known for their aggressive marketing tactics.

They may try to recast junk food as healthy food, and they often market right to children, who can't resist the siren call of an ad the way adults can. (Well, some adults, anyway!)

9. Misinformation

People who want to sell you something, like engineered food, have a vested interest in spreading some misinformation. However, they're not the only source. Many people in the media don't quite get the food and nutrition research right. Other times the data or the models are old or haven't yet been proven.

10. Some medications

You may be taking a prescription that leads to weight gain, such as some antidepressants known as SSRIs. Antipsychotics and some diabetes meds have the same effect. It's not that these medications have anything to do with willpower, but rather they cause changes in your body, such as increasing your appetite or lowering the metabolic rate at which energy is burned.

Age-related changes specific to women

As we mentioned earlier in the chapter, menopause is a stage in life for women with very distinct changes that can have an effect on their weight as well. You've already learned that you might go from a pear shape to an apple shape, but there are some additional reasons why women tend to put on weight at this stage.

You're losing muscle mass, and muscles burn more calories than fat. Eating the way you've always done and not changing your exercise will likely lead to weight gain just because of the muscle mass tissue.

However, you can fight menopause-related changes by reducing the excess weight you carry. Exercising or moving more will help, as can eating less. In your 50s, you may need roughly 200 fewer calories per day compared to your diet in the past couple of decades.[3] Watching your added sugars is also a good idea, as is drinking less alcohol and shoring up your support system. Not just for food-related issues, but to help reduce stress in general too.

There are some additional reasons women gain weight after age 40. Don't worry—none of these has to be your destiny as long as you change your lifestyle by following the plans later in the book.

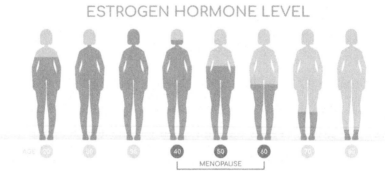

ESTROGEN HORMONE LEVEL

- Hormones

Estrogen and progesterone both take a dip in menopause now that the body no longer has to be concerned about getting pregnant. This can cause a dangerous amount of *visceral* fat to gather around your organs in your belly, and this type of fat is the one most associated with deadly conditions like cardiovascular disease and certain cancers.

The decrease in these hormones also leads to less bone density and decreases muscle mass. But it's not just about progesterone and estrogen hormones in menopause; enter the ghrelin and leptin hormones.

You already know that leptin tells the brain that you're full, but you might not know that ghrelin conversely tells the brain that you're hungry. When ghrelin is low, you're hungrier and end up wanting to eat more.

- Slower metabolism

Estrogen also plays a role in a slower metabolism, but your rate slows down and can hit a low during this time.

- Inactivity

As we grow older, we tend to be less active, at least here in the US, but we've got it exactly backward. Less activity means fewer calories burned, and the pounds start packing on.

It's important to start where you are. If you have a hard time walking around the block without getting out of breath, don't expect to get out there and run a five-mile race right away. If you have painful joints due to arthritis, you may not want to run at all, but water aerobics could be the right answer.

- Stress

Remember that you've got a brain that's still running on ancient hardware, and when we're stressed out, we're often in "fight-or-flight" mode. This raises the stress hormone cortisol. Periodic exposure to cortisol isn't actually bad for you—if you can calm back down by shaking it off, stress can actually help you focus.

However, modern life leads to a lot of cortisol because your routine day by day can be quite stressful. It's long-term cortisol exposure that's the problem, which can lead to added fat around the midsection.

Many women eat to try to soothe themselves, which leads to added pounds. We've included the mindfulness and dance chapters in the book to directly deal with the problem of stress.

- Lack of sleep

Modern life can also make it hard to sleep, which is a big problem. Not getting enough sleep may affect your hormones and your body's chemistry.

However, there's an even simpler problem. When you're tired, you want more energy. And the easiest way to get energy is to eat—after all, a calorie is a way to measure energy. But of course, that leads to excess weight as well.

Inspiration: Jennifer Lopez

If you're reading this book, then you may remember JLo all the way back when she was a Fly Girl on the hit TV show *In Living Color*. Of course, since then, she's been in a number of hit movies as well.

Despite her celebrity status, she's a woman who goes through the same age-related changes that we all do. But she's been able to continue looking fabulous as she grows older by making some lifestyle changes. You may not have the money to hire two personal trainers as she does, but then again, you're not followed by the paparazzi wherever you go!

In addition to her intense workouts, she also maintains a healthy and balanced eating plan. She gave up alcohol and caffeine years ago. A typical breakfast is a protein-packed shake, and lunch is a salad with lots of leafy greens. Fruits and veggies are good snacks for her, but she pairs them with nuts for more protein when she needs it.

Dinner is with the kids and consists of lean protein, veggies, and complex carbs like sweet potatoes or quinoa. And once a week, she allows herself dessert, so she doesn't have to feel deprived.

If you want to look like JLo and have a fabulous body like hers, it's a good idea to eat like her too.

Food for thought

Now you know about some of the things that are a result of the aging process…but many of them can be reversed.

- Are any of the symptoms of aging appearing in your own body?
- Do you feel more stressed than in your 20s and 30s?
- Are you taking steps now to increase your physical activity?
- What would you need to do in your life to make sure you get regular exercise if you're not doing it now?
- Who can you turn to for support as you begin your Whole Body journey?

Chapter Summary

There are a variety of things that happen to the human body as it grows older, but you don't have to be sick or overweight as you age. But once you're past the age of 40 or so, it's very easy to pack on the pounds unless you commit to better eating and nutrition, physical activity, and stress-reducing activities too.

---

1. https://medlineplus.gov/ency/article/003998.htm
2. https://www.healthline.com/nutrition/10-causes-of-weight-gain#TOC_TITLE_HDR_3
3. https://www.mayoclinic.org/healthy-lifestyle/womens-health/in-depth/menopause-weight-gain/art-20046058

IS MOVING YOUR BODY JUST AN "EXTRA" YOU CAN IGNORE?

"The only person you are destined to become is the person you decide to be."

— RALPH WALDO EMERSON

Many traditional books about losing weight focus on eating nutritiously and physical activity in the form of cardiovascular exercise like running or biking and resistance training or "lifting weights." They skimp on (or skip) the topic of stretching and may ignore dance entirely. Yet retaining flexibility as you age is key, and neither running nor lifting weights provides that benefit.

Later in the book, we'll go over specific stretches and dance workouts, but for right now you'll discover why it's so beneficial to incorporate these two into your physical movements. Forget the stretches that your 6th-grade gym teacher taught you in PE class—we're getting into the latest understanding of why stretching works and how to do it properly.

Why stretch?

If all those other books skip stretching, why can't you? In this book, we're concentrating on the science as we know it, and the science has come back heavily in favor of stretching.

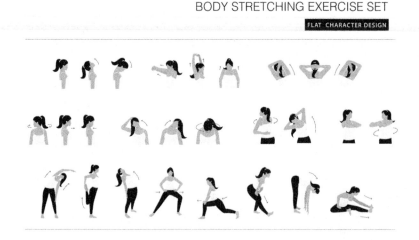

BODY STRETCHING EXERCISE SET
FLAT CHARACTER DESIGN

- Mobility and independence

Without keeping up your flexibility, it will be hard to move by yourself when you're older. You don't want to have to walk with a cane or a walker when you're trying to get from place to place. Being able to navigate steps right now might not seem like a big deal, but when your mobility is decreased, it will be.

The longer you can move about by yourself, the more independent you'll be as you grow older. You won't need as much help with simple things like climbing a few stairs, getting in and out of your car, and into and out of the grocery store.

- Maintain a wide range of motion in your joints

When your joints get tighter, it's hard to move around. Stretching can help keep your joints ready to do what they're supposed to do, which means you can stay active and mobile longer.

- Keeps muscles flexible

This flexibility also supports your joints having a better range of motion. If you're not stretching them, then they get weak and start to tighten up. Then when you need to use your muscles, it's hard for them to perform for you, and they can't extend all the way.

A good example is what sitting down does to your hamstrings, which are the big muscles at the back of your thighs. Staying seated all day is bad for you in general, but it also tightens up your hamstrings. Then it's harder for you to extend your legs all the way or straighten your knees. That makes it harder just to walk.

- Reduces your chances of getting injured

When your muscles are tight and then you use them suddenly, you might end up with injuries. This is why so-called "weekend warriors" tend to get hurt when they're exercising. They've been sitting all week and their muscles are tight, which leads to injury when they have to be stretched suddenly.

And injured muscles can't support the joints properly, which can lead to joint pain and damage as well. By contrast, healthy muscles that are regularly stretched are less susceptible to injury and can help prevent joint problems. In addition, having good muscle tone helps you keep your balance, so you're less likely to get hurt from a fall.

Best practices for stretching

It's best not to pay attention to the way you stretched two decades ago (if you stretched then) or the way that it's shown on movies and TV. There are ways to stretch that will help you reap all the benefits discussed above, and help you prevent overstretching or damaging yourself as you go.

- A warmup is a warmup, but stretching is not a warmup

If you haven't been moving around at all, then your muscles will be cold, and stretching them could mean injury. Research shows that stretching before an intense workout like sprinting or other explosive types of movement can actually make your hamstrings weaker.[1]

So rather than start off with your stretches, do a light warmup first for about five to ten minutes. In other words, do some easy walking, jogging, or biking first.

Or even better, stretch after your exercise. Then you know your muscles will be fully warmed up.

- Focus on major muscle groups

Don't worry so much about the smaller muscles—focus on the big groups instead. This includes your calves, hips, thighs, lower back, shoulders, and neck.

In addition, if there are other ones that you use on a regular basis, you should stretch those too. For example, if you work at a keyboard all day, you might want to stretch out your wrists.

Also, if you play sports, there are some sports-specific stretches that will probably benefit you. For instance, soccer players should stretch their hamstrings. Runners may need to stretch their feet too.

You don't need to push into pain when you're stretching - that means that you've gone too far. You should feel some tension, but not actual pain. If it does start to hurt, release the stretch and do one that doesn't feel so painful.

- Try to make moves symmetrical

Some people are born very flexible, and others aren't. If you couldn't be a gymnast when you were younger, you probably can't be that flexible now. Other people may be able to do the splits, but if you're just not that flexible, don't hurt yourself trying to do them.

In other words, your goal should be to be as flexible as your body can possibly be, even if you're nowhere near what other people are doing. It's also critical to try to be equally as flexible on both your right and left sides. Imbalance can mean injury. Many people tend to be more flexible on one side compared to each other but stretch to try to get your less flexible side more agile.

- Don't bounce

Once you've eased yourself into the stretch, avoid bouncing around in it. Just hold it, smoothly and evenly. Bouncing can actually cause some damage and potentially lead to more muscle tightness, not less.

- Hold for about one minute

For some stretches, this will feel like a long time. But as long as you've warmed up properly and you're not overstretching, you'll see the benefits. Also, remember to breathe while you're doing this!

- Be consistent and stretch at least three times a week

Just like other physical activity, doing this occasionally on a weekend isn't going to give you the positive results that you're hoping for. If you start increasing your range of motion by stretching, suddenly stopping could lead to a decrease in the range of motion.

It's a little bit like the principle of inertia: an object at rest tends to stay at rest. But an object in motion will keep moving, and you want to be an object in motion because that's what keeps you healthy.

Why dance workouts?

Maybe you were a dancer when you were younger and had dreams of being a ballerina. Or a Fly Girl, or a hip-hop star. On the other hand, maybe you stayed away from anything dance-related!

Either way, incorporating some dance workouts into your routine can help you be more flexible as well as burn some calories while you're enjoying your favorite music. Not only that, but learning new dance steps and new routines is good for your brain as you get older.

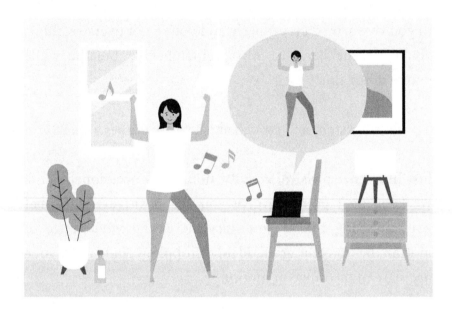

- Improved coordination

Because you're using different parts of your body when you dance, you build up your coordination. Now, you might not be able to start off with killer moves that young people will envy. But the more you learn dance steps that need coordination, the more coordinated you'll be.

If you're wondering why it's so important in middle age, improving your coordination doesn't just help you now, but in later life. You'll have better mobility when you can move smoothly. Plus coordination helps with your balance, which as you've learned can decline over time and lead to dangerous falls. Being better able to balance can help you avoid those falls.

- Better agility

Just like with stretching, being more agile protects your bones from harm as well as your muscles. When you get older, you'll be happy to be able to bend at the waist, hips, and knees. These movements are tough when you're inflexible and your joints have a hard time moving.

- More aerobic capacity

This is pretty much a fancy way of saying that dance is good for your heart. Because our culture focuses so much on women's breasts, you might not realize that breast cancer isn't even the most deadly cancer for women—lung cancer is. And yet, the top killer of both men and women is heart disease.[2]

Your heart is a muscle organ. Many people think of it as "just" an organ, but in fact, it's mostly cardiac muscle tissue. And like all muscles, the more you use it, the better off you are. That's why body movement is so critical for health.

Yes, exercise can help you maintain weight loss, but it's much more important than that. Your brain needs oxygenated blood to do its best work, and a dance routine is a fun way to keep your ticker pumping the way it's supposed to.

- Alter cholesterol levels

You've probably heard that cholesterol is bad, but your body makes it naturally. It's required to make healthy cells and generate vitamins and hormones. So you need some, but not too much.

It gets a little tricky because you often see just one number for cholesterol, but there are actually three different materials that make up your total cholesterol number.

1. HDL

This stands for high-density lipoprotein and is known as the "good" cholesterol because it removes the LDL from your arteries and carries it back to the liver, which can dispose of it. It can help protect against strokes and heart attacks, so you want a higher number for this one.

2. LDL

Low-density lipoprotein is the "bad" one because it's the one that can build up in your arteries. When they're narrower due to these buildups, it's harder for your blood to circulate the way it needs to. That increases the chances of having a heart attack or a stroke. You want a low LDL number.

3. Triglycerides

They store the excess energy (read: calories) from what you eat and are the most common type of fat in your body. They can contribute to the narrowing of your arteries if your LDL is too high or your HDL is too low. Like LDL, you need a low number of triglycerides for good health.

In a study, the dance routine was shown to increase the "good" cholesterol (HDL) and reduce triglycerides.[3] Which is another reason it's great for your heart.

• Improved brain health and memory

Learning keeps your brain young. Doing new things is great for your brain, especially as you grow older. Studies have shown that the brains of older dancers act younger than those of sedentary people.[4]

While many older people like to do crossword puzzles, which can help your brain as you grow older, dancing and learning new routines and steps gives you the added benefit of exercise and brainwork. Plus, if you take classes or go to a studio, you also have the benefit of being around other people, which helps combat loneliness.

Sounds great, right? Let's get dancing! However, you should follow a few practices as you begin incorporating dance into your routine.

Best practices for dancing

Yes, you can just load up a fun playlist and start moving and grooving to the beat! But if you haven't been dancing in a while, a few best practices will help you prevent injury. You may have been incredibly agile as a ballerina when you were 12, but you are no longer that flexible, and you'll hurt yourself if you try to dive back in where you left off. (This goes for other forms of dance as well.)

- Pick the style of dance you want

There are all kinds of different dances you can do! If you have a partner, you might want a style that works with couples (salsa and ballroom dancing comes to mind.) But you don't have to have a partner to dance.

And you don't have to do the same kind that you did as a kid (f you were a dancer back then). Just because you took ballet classes for years doesn't mean you can't do hip-hop now.

Choose something that feels good to you in terms of music and rhythm. If you hate classical music, then go for something more contemporary. If you haven't looked at dance workouts in a while, you might be surprised at all the varieties out there. This movement is just for you personally.

- Find classes or videos

To get started, especially if you're learning a new type of dance, taking classes can be very helpful. There are online classes, but as noted above, you also get a social benefit when you go to a physical dance class, so that might be an even better option. You're not going to be good at it at first, whether or not you danced when you were younger, so you don't have to worry about being graded or criticized.

If you're not a complete beginner, you might find that you can pick up a new style from an online video. There are plenty, so don't worry about finding them.

- Go easy at first

If you haven't been dancing for a while, you will not be starting at the same level as where you left off a decade or two ago. Give yourself a break. You may have some muscle memory that starts coming back, but you probably don't have the agility or speed that you did back then.

Don't expect to pick things up immediately. Ease into it, and maybe try a little easier style of dance when you're first dipping your toe into the dancing waters. Going hard up front and all the time is a recipe for injury, so protect your body and be gentle to it.

- Warmup

Getting your heart rate up with a little light walking or jogging can warm your legs up so they're better able to handle the dance. Just like with stretching, starting cold is a bad idea. Remember legwarmers in the 80s? Dancers use them for a reason—to protect their valuable leg muscles from getting too cold.

Warming up helps your tendons and ligaments to loosen up a bit as well, which will also help prevent injury.

- How do you get to Carnegie Hall?

Practice, practice, practice! Even if you're not trying to memorize a dance routine (though don't forget, that's good for your brain!), being consistent about the time you spend dancing is a good idea.

You don't have to be consistent in the type of dance you do. Maybe one day you feel like doing a more ballet-oriented dance, and then a couple of days later, it's all about the line dance. It doesn't really matter whether you stick with one or try a number of different types of routines, as long as you change it up every so often so your mind can get a workout too.

Mostly, adding a dance habit should feel good in your body and your mind. Music that you enjoy can help you express your feelings through dance too. There really aren't any rules (except the ones you read above!), so just get out there and get your groove back.

Inspiration: Sharon Stone

She may have been young when she exploded onto the scene in the movie *Basic Instinct*, but decades later, in her 60s, she's still fit and sexy. She likes to mix it up (remember that novelty is excellent for the aging brain!) and includes dance routines in her workouts.

Food for thought

Now that you've learned how important stretching and dance are once you reach middle age and beyond, think about how you can incorporate these into your life.

- Do you know which parts of your body tend to be tight and which tend to be more flexible?
- Which side is more flexible than the other?
- How often can you commit to a series of stretching exercises?
- What kinds of music do you like to move to?
- Is there a type of dance you like to do or have always wanted to learn more about?
- Would you prefer to go to a studio or stay in the comfort of your own home to dance?

Chapter Summary

Stretching and dance are good for your brain and your body. The key to both is to start where you are right now and not go too hard too soon. That could lead to injury. Instead, begin with what you can do now and when you can add it to your routine, and then build from there.

———————————————

1. https://www.mayoclinic.org/healthy-lifestyle/fitness/in-depth/stretching/art-20047931
2. https://www.cdc.gov/heartdisease/facts.htm
3. https://www.eatthis.com/news-dancing-exercise-menopause/
4. https://www.eatthis.com/news-side-effect-dancing/

YOUR KEY TO FOOD MASTERY: THE 10 RULES OF CLEAN EATING

"A year from now you may wish you'd started today."

— KAREN LAMB

In the previous chapter, we discussed the physical movement aspect of getting to and maintaining a healthy weight: stretching and dance. However, you can't out-dance a bad diet, and that's where healthy eating comes in.

Because of our culture's emphasis on exercise, many people believe that they can lose weight by exercise alone. But for the vast majority of Americans, that's just not true.[1]

However, you can see the needle on the scale start heading in the right direction when you combine a good eating plan with exercise.

You've discovered the benefits of physical movement. Even if exercise alone doesn't move the needle, it still benefits you in a variety of ways. Similarly, a way of eating known as *clean eating* has a multitude of upsides for your health. One caveat, though: you should see your doctor to make sure you don't have any health issues you need to resolve before starting clean eating—just to be on the safe side!

What is clean eating?

You might have heard of it but do not know exactly what it is. One thing that I want to make clear here is that clean eating is not a diet in terms of a weight loss program that you "go on," like paleo or keto or any kind of name-brand diet. That's because they don't work in the long run.[2]

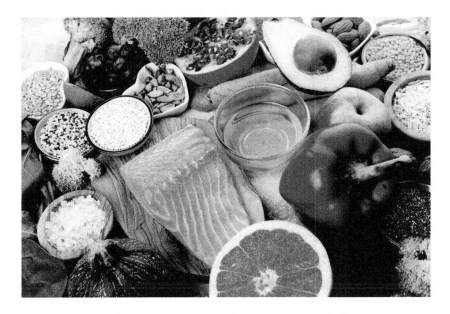

People often have success at first, because they're motivated to get started and find it easy to buy the "right" foods. But over time, if they haven't made a change to their lifestyle, they stop buying the food, or it becomes inconvenient as they're less motivated. And then the pounds creep right back on.

Instead, clean eating is a way of eating that will serve you for the rest of your life. You'll be eating nutritious foods that your body recognizes as food, and you'll feel more satisfied with your meals and less deprived. In conjunction with the mindset changes that we'll explore in a later chapter, plus the body movement, you'll have no need to binge on sugar or other comfort foods, or "eat your feelings" as so many Americans do.

The definition of clean eating that we're using here means that you're eating foods as close to their natural state as possible, without additional preservatives or additives. You'll be choosing foods that are free from refined and processed ingredients.

Think about your grocery store. Most of them are organized along similar lines: fruits and vegetables, dairy, eggs, and fresh meat and fish tend to be on the perimeter of the store. If you shop at more than one store, you'll probably still find those categories of food on the perimeter.

What's in the middle of the store, in the aisles? All the processed food, such as processed deli meats, ice cream, frozen chicken nuggets or fish sticks, ready-to-eat mixes, macaroni and cheese boxes and pouches, and the like. They contain artificial ingredients designed to make them "shelf-stable." Many of these products include types of fats (trans fats) that are known to promote heart disease.

As a clean eater, you'll do most of your shopping around the perimeter, not in the aisles. However, a few ingredients, such as nuts and beans, are usually found on the inside of the store and are excellent for clean eaters.

This type of food plan does require more cooking and fewer trips to go out to eat since many restaurants also have food packed with additives and preservatives. But don't worry; even though you'll be making meals from scratch, there are ways to speed up the meal planning and prep process. It doesn't actually take much more time than if you decided to order takeout and wait for the delivery driver or go to the restaurant yourself.

Whole foods around the perimeter of the store tend to have more vitamins and minerals present because the act of processing food generally removes them from the food. Sometimes they're added back in, but it may not be in a form that your body can easily use. (And why spend the additional money to buy processed food with the vitamins added back in when you could just buy the real thing?)

In addition to reducing your reliance on over-processed foods, clean eating will help you reduce the sodium in your meals as well as sugar. Many boxed and frozen meals include heaping helpings of both salt and sugar to convince you to keep coming back for more. While your body does need some salt, it doesn't need a lot, and it really doesn't need added sugar at all. You'll also be drinking fewer sugary drinks on your clean eating plan.

These whole foods are nutrient-dense, so your body will be able to function potentially without any additional supplements. They have plenty of vitamins, minerals, higher-quality protein, and fats that support your health. Fat-free diets were popular in the 1990s and still are in some circles, but your body actually needs good fats to function optimally. You'll discover what these fats are a bit later in the book.

Clean eating focuses on whole grains, good protein and fats, and fruits and vegetables that your body recognizes and can use for good health.

All of this may sound good, but are there additional benefits to clean eating besides avoiding fillers and artificial ingredients?

Benefits of eating clean

Not everything artificial is bad, and not everything natural is good. (After all, the hemlock that Socrates used to kill himself was all natural!) However, when it comes to food, eating whole foods that are as close to their natural state and unprocessed as possible does have distinct advantages for your health.

- Better heart health

Good fats and nutrition help prevent the onset of inflammation, which is known to cause cardiovascular disease. Whole, unprocessed foods support your heart instead of causing fatty plaques to form. These fatty plaques can break off in the arteries and form clots that may cause heart attacks or strokes.

- Better brain health

Tired of brain fog? Eat clean! You're feeding your brain the nutrients it needs for optimal function.

- Stronger immune system

Your body tries to protect itself from processed food and excess sugar, which means there's not much of your immune system left over to fight against bacteria, viruses, and other attackers. Once your immune system can focus on what it needs to pay attention to, you'll have a stronger immune response which can better help you fight off diseases.

- Decreased inflammation

Many health conditions and diseases have their roots in inflammation. You've probably heard of it, but many people don't know exactly what it is. It's the body's protective response to anything that could injure it.

Acute inflammation isn't dangerous, and it happens when you bang against something or cut yourself. The body sends out white blood cells to surround and protect the area while it's healing, which results in swelling and redness.

It's chronic inflammation that's the problem, and it's the response to unwanted materials in the body, like the toxins inhaled from cigarette smoke or too much fat. But when you're eating clean, there are fewer substances for your body to protect you from, and so you have less inflammation.

- Increased energy

The problem with caffeine, sugar, energy drinks, and the like, is that they're temporary fixes. You might get an immediate energy rush, but it's likely followed by a nasty energy crash. When you're eating clean and you don't need to rely on these fast but unreliable substances, you'll have more energy on a consistent basis.

Plus, you'll be better able to sleep at night because your system isn't trying to digest food that it has problems with. Which leads to more energy as well.

- Improved skin

Who doesn't want their face to have a healthy glow? When you're eating clean and absorbing more vitamins, minerals, and nutrients, it helps boost all the processes that give you better skin and nails.

- Sunnier moods

You might not hear about this from the makers of antidepressants, but there is a strong connection between the food you eat and how good you feel, which can put you in a better mood.

Think about the times you remember being in a good mood, for whatever reason. How did your body feel? Lumpy and heavy, as it often does after you've eaten a big fast food meal? Probably not—you likely felt light and full of energy, which is what clean eating can give you.

Not only that, but sugar is a well-known mood alterer. Removing excess sugar from your diet can help you avoid the mood swings linked to sugar.

- More willpower

If you've ever tried to take sugar out of your diet, you know that the first few days are the hardest—but then your sugar cravings seem to magically disappear! By eating clean you won't be subject to the same physical cravings that make it hard to stick to an eating plan.

And because there are so many yummy foods and recipes that go along with clean eating, you won't feel deprived. So you won't have the same mental cravings either.

These benefits probably sound pretty great. But which foods exactly will bring you all these advantages?

The 10 golden rules of clean eating

The good news is that while there are some foods (or "foods") to avoid, there are plenty of great-tasting ones that you can add to your diet when you're eating clean. One way to feel less deprived is to focus on what you can eat as opposed to what you can't.

Eating clean is also pretty simple: it's not like you can only eat one type of berry and not another, for example. You can eat them all! Making the plan simple will help you stick to it, and it won't be so hard to remember what to get at the grocery store.

  1. Skip processed foods that contain sugar, preservatives, and artificial coloring

When you think about it, processed food takes a long time to get from the farm to your pantry. It has to make it through processing, then transported to the grocery store, and then into your home. That means it's chock full of preservatives to ensure that it lasts all that time and remains shelf-stable.

Some estimates say that Americans eat over 1,000 *billion* pounds of chemical food additives per year![3] That's a lot, especially when you consider that the laws regulating these chemicals are pretty lax.

Additives can have a variety of negative effects on the body. Artificial flavoring, for instance, has been linked to behavioral problems. The pesticides, antibiotics, and hormones used in farming (for plants and meat) are associated with ADHD and Parkinson's disease, among other conditions.

By eating fresh, whole foods, you won't need any preservatives or other additives, so you won't have to deal with the negative consequences either.

2. Avoid refined sugars

You already know what sugar is but not be quite so clear on refined sugar. Sugar occurs naturally in fruits and vegetables but also in dairy, grains, seeds, and nuts. When you eat a piece of cheese or a strawberry, you do get the naturally occurring sugar such as fructose or lactose, but you also get all the nutrients and vitamins and minerals from the food.

There are two main refined sugars that you'll come across in packaged foods (including candy)—sucrose (table sugar) and high-fructose corn syrup or HFCS. These are the kinds that you want to avoid. Refined sugars are linked to excess belly fat, obesity, type 2 diabetes, and heart disease.

The foods that typically have a lot of refined sugars are also heavily processed (therefore violating rule #1 as well). If you look at the label, in addition to seeing the names sugar, cane sugar, HFCS, molasses, rice syrup, or other clear signals of sugar, you might also see chemicals that end in "ose," such as maltose or dextrose. That means sugar, so put that container with the label back on the shelf.

Expect to see it in a number of aisles at the grocery store: not just baked goods but canned beans, pretty much anything labeled "low-fat," ketchup, pizza, breakfast bars, muesli, and energy and "sport" drinks.

3. Miss out on white foods

Maybe you're wondering what's so bad about white foods, by which I mean white rice, white bread, white sugar, and so forth. Think about what whole foods you know that are white. There are only a few fruits and vegetables that are truly white, and a few fish.

But other than that, whole foods tend to be colorful. Brown is generally the color for sugar, rice, and whole grains. But you can find the entire rainbow in fruits and vegetables: red, orange, yellow, green, blue, and violet abound.

White foods, therefore, were probably processed from some other food. White rice has the most nutritious part removed, which gives it a white color. Similarly, white bread is made from white flour, which in turn started out as brown grains that had their nutritious parts removed to get the white color.

You've already learned how dangerous processed food can be, which is why the third golden rule is to stay away from white foods that have been processed. (But feel free to eat your white asparagus, turnips, and other fruits and vegetables that happen to be white!)

4. No refined carbohydrates

Please notice that we're not saying you should avoid all carbs because you shouldn't. Just the specific type that is worse for your health.

What is a carbohydrate anyway? It's a macronutrient or energy source for the body, and it's actually a sugar molecule. The body breaks this molecule down into glucose, which is the type of sugar that it runs on. It can either be used right away or stored inside your liver and muscles.

Sugars and simple carbs are found not only in candy and cake but in fruit, milk, etc. Starches are complex carbs, which means they're made of multiple sugar molecules. They include bread and pasta as well as peas, corn, and potatoes.

Fiber is also a complex carb, and most of these carbs can't be broken down by your body. That helps you feel fuller so you don't have to eat as much. They're found mostly in plant-based foods like fruits and vegetables, grains, seeds, and nuts.

If you're eating whole foods, then you're getting the carbs closest to their natural state when it comes to nuts and seeds, fruits, and veggies. You should also try minimally processed items like bread, which will be made from grains that haven't had the nutrients removed.

The main sources of refined carbs are the ones that can promote obesity, type-2 diabetes, and heart disease. You might recall these are linked to refined sugar, and that's one of the most common refined carbs. The other is refined grains, which you see in white bread and food like boxed cake and cookie mixes.

Refined carbs are found in many of the foods that you can buy at the grocery store, including soda and other beverages. You might have noticed that many of these categories avoid overlapping each other.

They're found in prepackaged mixes and condiments and sodas and all the other foods that you typically find in the middle of the store. If you toss something back because it violates the first rule, chances are high it'll violate two, three, and four as well.

5. Include plenty of protein

Protein is one of the three macronutrients, and it's easy to get from the standard American diet. You'll feel fuller longer when you're getting enough protein because it takes longer for the body to break down. Proteins are made from amino acids, and nine of them are necessary for good health, but your body doesn't make it on its own.

The recommended minimum is 0.36 grams of protein per pound of body weight. If you weigh 140 pounds, you'll need about 50 grams a day. But if you're active, pregnant, or breast-feeding—or even an older adult—you'll need more than that.

It's necessary while you're eating clean, but you'll need to look for higher quality sources than what you might be used to eating. Many people automatically think of beef and chicken and other animal sources, but don't forget yogurt (especially the Greek style, which is strained), eggs, almonds, lentils, quinoa, beans, and pumpkin seeds.

6. Eat organic fruits and vegetables

Organic farms don't use pesticides. Since pesticides are linked to a number of negative outcomes, I recommend eating organic instead. Only natural fertilizers are allowed (to be certified organic), and weeds are managed through natural means like crop rotation and hand-pulling instead of synthetic herbicides (though organic ones are approved).

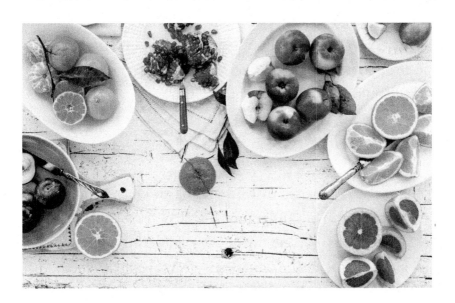

Natural methods like birds, bugs, and traps are used to deal with pests instead of pesticides. Although companies have developed all kinds of chemicals to deal with farms, it's also possible to use the old, natural ways too. The natural methods are often better for nearby animals and people.

Organic farming tends to be better for the environment as well. It can help conserve water, reduce pollution and soil erosion, and even make the soil better for growing.

You may have heard people talk about "eating local," which means you eat from local farms and generally eat what's in season. Your nearest farmer's market is a great place to start.

However, bear in mind that certification for organic food is expensive, and not all family farms can afford it. They may still use organic practices. So don't ignore a stall that doesn't have the certification: you want a farm that practices it, and a piece of paper doesn't matter. Ask the person at the stall how they handle pests, fertilizer, etc.

7. Don't forget whole grains

Due to the popularity of keto and paleo diets, some people are unwilling to add in grains. But they provide fiber and B vitamins like niacin and folate, as well as other minerals such as zinc, iron, and magnesium. Don't ignore them just because bread has such as bad reputation!

It's important to avoid refined grains, as you read earlier. A whole grain has all three of its parts intact. The bran, which is the outer layer, contains most of the fiber, as well as a little B vitamin and protein. The endosperm, which is the next layer down, contains carbs and a little protein and vitamins and minerals. The germ, or the seed inside, has more B and E vitamins and minerals.

Plenty of whole grains other than whole wheat flour, rolled oats, and brown rice are easy to cook up and don't need a lot of preservatives to sit in your pantry for a little while. Whole grains contribute to friendly bacteria in your gut, which help you digest food properly and also benefit your heart, brain, skin, and mood!

Now you know why you need to include them. Americans are relatively unfamiliar with many grains such as amaranth (not technically a grain, but treated like one in cooking) and barley, which tends to be chewy and has a pleasantly nutty flavor.

Buckwheat, like amaranth, isn't technically a grain. Toast or roast it before cooking with it to really bring out its flavor.

There are different ways to use wheat than you might be accustomed to. Wheat "berries" are the whole grain. Bulgur, or cracked wheat, is the whole grain cracked and partially cooked. Freekeh is green, young cracked wheat. There's also farro, which can refer to several different varieties of hulled wheat: einhorn, emmer, and spelt.

All of those wheat varieties can be a problem for those who have been diagnosed with celiac disease. If you have celiac, and even if you don't, you can also try millet, which is an ancient type of grain, or quinoa and its cousin, kaniwa. Teff, another ancient grain, could also be a good choice. It's from Ethiopia and is often used in their bread injera.

8. Cook with healthy oils and fats

Unfortunately, the fat-free craze of the 1990s left a lot of people overweight because it simply replaced fats with sugar. Also, fat is the third micronutrient, and you do need some in your diet for good health.

The issue is avoiding fats and oils that have been processed in such a way that they're dangerous to your health. They're often known as trans fats, and these you should steer clear of. Saturated fats and oils may contribute to high cholesterol, so minimize them—these are typically animal fats like dairy, beef, and coconut and palm oils.

When you're thinking about cooking oils, it's important to consider the smoke point at which the oil burns and begins to break down, releasing free radicals that contribute to inflammation and some other chemicals.

Great oils that are minimally processed and have a smoke point high enough for most cooking include olive oil, which is good for baking; avocado oil, which has a higher smoke point and is good for frying, and sesame oil and safflower oils, which similarly have a high smoke point.

Avoid palm oil in your cooking because it's unsustainable. Walnut and flax oils are healthy but not for cooking—leave them for your salad dressings.

Because fat has more calories per gram than either carbs or protein, you don't want to eat too much of it. Good sources of fats include avocados, fish, nuts, and seeds.

9. Snack on nuts

These tasty snacks come from seed kernels. They are rich in nutrients, as you discovered above, since they contain fiber, protein, and fat! They tend to be high in calories due to all the fat content, so you don't need too much at any time—just one ounce of whichever one you feel like.

They also contain plenty of antioxidants, which fight inflammation and too many free radicals in the body. (It turns out your body does need some free radicals!) They've been shown to help people lose weight, in addition to lowering cholesterol, including triglyceride levels.[4] They're good for your heart and may lower your chances of having a heart attack or stroke.

Nuts are best either raw or toasted, without oils. Dry roasting is your next best bet. While you can leave them in your pantry at room temperature, they'll last longer if you keep them in the freezer.

10. Choose beans

Lentils and beans, along with peanuts and peas, are legumes. They're low in fat and higher in protein, in addition to being a good source of certain vitamins and minerals. Beans are eaten all over the world due to their versatility, but many Americans could benefit from adding more of them into their meals.

Beans have a lot of soluble fiber, so they help protect your heart and your weight loss goals. They fill you up faster, so you're not as hungry. Typically they also contain a lot of iron, so they're a good choice for anyone who tends to be anemic. Because they're digested more slowly, they also help prevent blood sugar spikes.

And they're the least expensive form of protein available. They can also be the most convenient, as you can find them in bulk, dried, canned, or even ground. Just beware the canned varieties as they tend to contain a lot of salt. Drain and rinse thoroughly to reduce the salt.

Are you going to obey these rules every single day? No, of course not. (Even our clean eating inspiration below, Gwyneth Paltrow, eats off her plan from time to time.) The key is to eat clean *most of the time*. You're going to end up at parties where you want an adult beverage or a slice of cake or whatever. During the holidays, you might want to indulge in your favorite treat. Just keep them to moderate portion sizes, and don't feel guilty about enjoying it. Your next meals will be clean.

Too many people have all-or-nothing thinking when it comes to food or meal plans. "Well, I messed up and had a cookie at lunch, so might as well have some pizza and ice cream for dinner!" Instead, think about treats that you genuinely love and make space for them occasionally. Allow yourself to have fun at the party!

All you have to do is eat clean most of the time. Just because you didn't eat clean at one meal doesn't mean all is lost. After all, when you dent your car, do you decide "the heck with it" and then total it? Don't total your plan for eating clean after you dent it by eating some processed foods, either.

Inspiration: Gwyneth Paltrow

Gwyneth Paltrow is an actor known especially for her star turn in the film *Shakespeare in Love*. She founded her own wellness empire, Goop, and has remained fit and in good health well into middle age.

She loves clean eating and talks about its benefits a lot. Hers is mostly vegan, but you don't have to go that far if you don't want to. (And if you do? Go for it!) She typically starts her day off with a healthy smoothie and has protein and salad for lunch. Generally, she eats whatever she wants for dinner and indulges in French-style desserts and adult beverages from time to time as well.

Food for thought

Now that you're clear on what clean eating means, you can look at what you've been eating to see what will work for your body.

- Do you have symptoms of inflammation or other issues caused by a bad diet?
- Have you been on a diet plan that didn't let you eat certain foods that you can now allow back in?
- What healthy foods have you been skipping that you can add to your meals?
- Are there new foods you hadn't heard about that you're excited to try?
- What's in your house that you should get rid of because they don't belong on a clean eating plan?

Chapter Summary

Whole, unprocessed foods are healthier, and many keep you fuller longer so you can eat less. It's important to recognize that occasional treats are perfectly fine. Just make most of your meals clean and you'll start reaping the benefits.

---

1. https://www.healthline.com/health-news/exercise-good-for-you-but-does-it-help-weight-loss#Exercise-doesn't-always-lead-to-weight-loss
2. https://www.healthline.com/health-news/diets-work-for-one-year#How-to-fight-back
3. https://www.theconsciouschallenge.org/ecologicalfootprint-bibleoverview/food-chemicals

4. https://www.healthline.com/nutrition/8-benefits-of-nuts#

DETOX DYNAMITE

"**Our bodies are our gardens - our wills are our gardeners.**"

— WILLIAM SHAKESPEARE

Y ou've got the ideal foods for your new lifestyle. You could go shopping and start on the meal plans right away. Yet even better, plan to detox first. It's a key piece of separating from your old ways and getting started with the new.

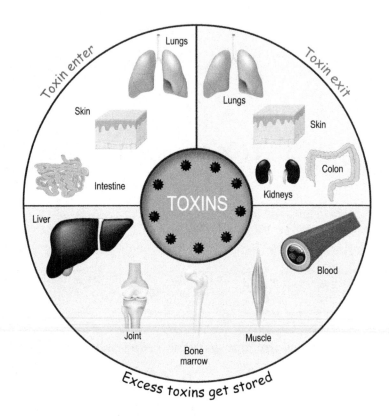

What does it mean to detox?

Detoxification isn't just a buzzword or the latest fad. It's the process of ridding your body of materials that are toxic to it. Of course, your body is already very good at detoxifying itself: your liver, kidneys, lungs, digestive tract, and even your skin help you release toxins.

Now you might be asking, what do I need detox for if detox diets don't do anything? The answer is that your body does the best job when each of those organs is healthy. If you've been eating a traditional American diet and not exercising, your body isn't necessarily able to handle getting rid of all the toxins that it encounters.

A properly designed detox (that doesn't involve dangerous laxatives or diuretics) can help your body optimize for detoxification. There are a number of ideas to incorporate into your detox.

- Maximize your sleep

Your mom (or grandma) might have told you to get enough sleep, and she was right. The brain and body do a lot of work when you're asleep that they can't do when you're awake. The brain is processing learning from the day and strengthening neural pathways or pruning them back as appropriate. Cells flush waste, and your body builds muscle.

When you don't get enough sleep, you're groggy and can't think as well the next day. Plus, you're more liable to get sick because your immune system is down when you're not getting sleep. Not only that, but your body wants energy, so you may be eating more and having cravings for sugary foods because those provide quicker hits of energy.

Each sleep cycle has three to four stages (one stage is usually for when you're dozing off, so you may only experience that once per night.) Different sleep stages provide different benefits, so they're all important. And your body needs to cycle through all the stages several times a night to get everything done.

In general, most adults need 7–8 hours of sleep, which allows you to cycle through all the sleep stages several times. People who are very active, like endurance athletes, often need more sleep. And you may find during your detox that you feel refreshed after more sleep as well.

Having trouble sleeping? The three magic words for a bedroom conducive to sleep are cool, dark, and quiet. Do not bring your phone into your bedroom, much less into your bed. The light tricks your body into thinking it's daytime, plus you're not accomplishing anything late at night except maybe stressing yourself needlessly. If you need an alarm, buy an alarm clock.

Ceiling fans can help cool off the room if you don't like a hefty air-conditioning bill, especially in the summer. You can buy room-darkening window fixtures or wear a sleep mask to make it dark enough. If your room or neighborhood is loud, a white noise machine or earplugs can help.

Many Americans, especially in middle age, find themselves ruminating over the day late at night. Stop the thoughts running around your head by writing in a journal, doing yoga, or meditating at the end of the day.

- Limit (or skip) alcohol

The old wisdom was that women could have one alcoholic drink a day and men two, but now it looks like a safe amount of alcohol is really closer to zero. Too much drinking is bad for your liver, which is one of the key organs in the body's detox system. Don't weigh it down with too much booze.

- Decrease the sugar, salt, and processed foods

All of these foods can stress the body and cause inflammation when you eat too much, as you discovered in the last chapter. Reducing the amount of junk food you eat makes it much easier for your liver and kidneys to do their jobs.

If you're feeling bloated from too much salt, drinking more water will help. So will adding some potassium-rich whole foods like squash, potatoes, bananas, spinach, and kidney beans.

- Drink enough water

The human body needs plenty of water in order to function at its best. It helps your body regulate its temperature, helps with digestion, lubricates your joints, and helps carry away waste products for detoxification. Roughly three liters a day is great for many people, depending on your activity level and where you live.[1]

One of the easiest ways to take in less sugar is to simply switch all your sodas to water instead. If you don't like the taste of water, you can buy filters or different kinds of bottled water. (Don't get plastic bottles, they just destroy the environment.) Some people don't like cold water, so if that's you, leave it at room temperature. Don't like it warm? Put it in the fridge!

You can add taste without calories or sugar. Infuse your water with fruits and vegetables or squeeze a lemon or lime in it. Keep a BPA-free reusable bottle with you so you always have water and aren't tempted to grab a soda.

- Eat foods with lots of antioxidants and prebiotics

You've probably heard of these terms, though what they mean exactly might not be clear. Antioxidants, which occur naturally in many whole foods, fight the stress on the body that's generated by free radicals. These molecules are missing an electron, and so they may "steal" an electron from somewhere else.

Your body generates some free radicals in its own processes, including digestion. And you don't want to get rid of all the free radicals. But the dose is the poison, and too many of these molecules play a part in diseases like Alzheimer's, heart and liver disease, and some types of cancer.

Antioxidants are plentiful in whole foods, especially fruits and vegetables. You've heard "eat the rainbow," and that makes sense because all the different colors come from different kinds of antioxidants: the orange in carrots comes from beta-carotene, for example. Antioxidants also include vitamins E, C, and A. It's better to get them from food and not from supplements.

Prebiotics are what come before probiotics, which are the good bacteria in your gut that aid in digestion and support the immune system. Yogurt and other fermented foods have plenty of probiotics. Prebiotics come in the form of fiber, which feeds the probiotics. Onions, garlic, asparagus, tomatoes, artichokes, bananas, and oats are all good sources of prebiotics.

- Get active

Exercise reduces inflammation and helps your body function properly, including the detoxification system. Plus, as we discussed earlier, it makes you feel good.

Reasons to detox

Still not sure why a natural detox can help you? We've got plenty of reasons you should give yourself a detox for your whole body reset.

1. You'll feel better

So many Americans in mid-life just don't feel very good. You might have aches and pains or be unhappy with the way you look with all the extra weight. And your body probably doesn't love how it feels with all the extra weight, either.

Those foods that you've previously been eating may make you feel sluggish, so getting rid of them will boost your energy naturally. Getting rid of them often helps people improve their skin as well, so they look better in the mirror.

2. You'll get rid of cravings

Eliminating adding sugar can help stop cravings. You may take a few days to get through it, but then you'll notice that you no longer crave sugar. It causes your brain to release dopamine and opioids or feel-good chemicals, which is why it may take a few days before the cravings stop.

This is where a clean eating plan can really help you because many processed foods, even ones you don't think taste very sweet, come loaded with sugar. Even ketchup has lots of sugar in it, so you need to be careful about what you're buying to make sure you're truly avoiding the sugar.

By avoiding processed foods, including sodas, sports, and energy drinks, you'll be removing a lot of sugar from your diet.

3. You can eliminate sensitivities

Toxins often trigger allergic reactions, so removing them from your body and making your body better able to deal with them means you might get some significant allergy relief. The detox reduces the load on your body's systems, which makes it easier to filter the allergens in your blood. In turn, that makes it easier for your immune system to function.

You may eliminate certain foods from your meals during the detox and see how you fare without them. Then when you add them back in (one by one) and experience a flare-up, you know you're sensitive to that food and should probably stop eating it.

4. Your sex life may improve

One consequence of not feeling good and not liking what you see in the mirror is often a lower sex drive. You don't want other people seeing or being intimate with your naked body. Detoxing can often help with your hormones, which might be flagging due to inflammation and excess weight.

What you might not realize is that having a lot of anxiety can also decrease your libido.[2] Later in the book, we'll discuss some mindfulness tools, but getting more sleep and journaling could be a step in the right direction.

5. Your digestion will be better

You guessed it—removing toxins and substances that are hard on the body also makes the process of digestion much easier on your stomach and intestines. Eating unprocessed food and washing them down with lots of water reduces the load on your body.

6. You'll be sharper

Feeling foggy and unfocused? Extra weight, inflammation, not moving much, and too much junk food can definitely make you feel like you can't think very well. These contaminants cause issues in the body, and so resources are diverted away from your brain, heart, and other muscles that require a lot of energy.

By getting rid of pollutants in your body and allowing your body to better eliminate them, the resources can be redirected back to your brain. More oxygenated blood flow and less inflammation add up to clearing out the brain fog.

7. You'll lose weight

You already know the benefits of losing weight when you've got too much extra padding. By reducing your intake of sugary, salty, and processed foods, you'll probably be reducing calories right off the bat, as long as you eat reasonable portions of the whole foods we've discussed.

Inspiration: Demi Moore

She's been in many movies stretching all the way back to the 1980s, and even after three kids she's kept her shape and stayed fit. Although she's been through some rough patches when she struggled with her body image, she's now at peace with her body and appreciates all it does for her.

She follows a raw vegan diet, which focuses on organic, clean eating. She dines on whole grains and plenty of protein, eating when she's hungry and stopping when she's full. (She also continues to work on her flexibility in addition to strength at the gym!)

While raw vegan food is not necessary or even optimal for everybody, you can take her approach with its emphasis on whole and organic foods, as well as being mindful while she's eating.

Food for thought

- Are you ready to improve your body's detoxification processes?
- Which of the reasons for a detox most speaks to you?
- Do you need to make adjustments to get the sleep you need?
- Are you currently missing out on antioxidants and prebiotics?
- If you don't currently drink enough water, what's your plan to make sure you drink more?

Chapter Summary

A healthy, natural detox helps your body's natural detoxification systems run better. Getting your body a detox jump start provides many different benefits.

---

1. https://www.healthline.com/nutrition/how-to-detox-your-body#3.-Drink-more-water
2. https://longevitylive.com/sex/detox-sex-life/

5

STRETCHING FOR YOUR LIFE

"Exercise is king. Nutrition is queen. Put them together and you've got a kingdom."

— JACK LALANNE

There are plenty of different stretches that can help you become more flexible and stay that way as you age. So if you have a favorite stretch for a specific part of the body, you can swap it in. Or you might want to try all new stretches to help mix it up a little bit. We'll get into the specifics of stretching for the 14-day reset in this chapter. You may find you want to continue them after the reset as well!

Remember to warm up before you stretch, with a little walking or light jogging, and maybe some arm waving when you get to the upper body stretches. Trying to stretch cold muscles is a recipe for injury. Be gentle with your body and start where you are. Also, make sure you hold the stretch for 30–60 seconds without bouncing. If you can't quite do the stretch for a whole minute, then start with 30 seconds and work your way up.

If you haven't been stretching in a long time, you won't be very flexible, so don't expect it. If it hurts or you feel a sharp pain, you've gone too far. What you should feel is some tension and maybe tightness, but no aches and pains.

Some people are physically limited in their flexibility, and if you're one of them, be mindful of how far you can go. Maybe you'll never be as flexible as your friend who can do the splits. That's okay. You need your body to be as agile as it can be, so stretch to your own limits and not someone else's. Everybody is different, and yours is the only one to be concerned about.

Leg and hip stretches

As mentioned earlier, starting off with stretches for the bigger muscles will really help your flexibility.

1. Standing hamstring stretch

Your hamstrings are the big muscles on the backs of your thighs. They're the ones that help you bend your knees and lift your leg straight out behind you. Hamstrings help you walk, run, do squats, and climb stairs. As you can see, they'll be pretty important for you in old age since they'll keep you mobile.

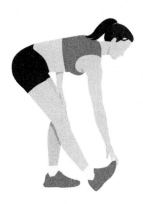

Do this stretch gently because when you're standing to stretch these muscles, you'll be making a deep stretch. Ease into it to make sure that you're not stretching too far.

- From a standing position, lift one heel and put it on the edge of a slightly higher surface, like a stair or curb.
- Keep your back straight as you bend at the hips, so your chest is close to your thigh. Your other knee will bend a bit too. Hold this pose.
- After you've stretched one leg, switch to the other one.

The key here is to keep your back straight and not round it. That can be hard, especially if your hamstrings are tight. You have to fold from the hips to stretch these muscles and avoid injuring your back fully.

If your hips or hamstrings are tight, that probably means you won't be able to fold as far forward. You might only be able to tilt a few inches, and that's fine. As you increase your flexibility, you'll be able to fold a little farther. It's progress, not perfection.

As always, when stretching both sides, you'll probably find that one side is easier than the other. Make sure you're holding the stretch for the same amount of time on each side —don't give up on your less flexible side too soon.

Make it easier: wall hamstring stretch

- Lie down at a wall corner or near a sofa.
- Leave one leg straight and lift the other against the wall or sofa.

- Push your knee as straight as you can and hold it.

2. Figure 4

This stretch is excellent for those with tight hips. It can also help stretch out your glutes or the muscles underneath your butt. You do it lying down, which often feels nice, especially after you've warmed up.

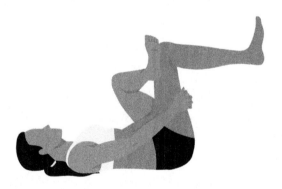

- Lie on your back with your feet flat on the floor and knees bent.
- Cross your right foot over your left knee. Keep your right foot flexed (instead of pointed).

- Bring your left knee towards your chest, with the right foot sitting on it. Then reach through your legs to lace your fingers together just under the back of your knee.
- Pull your left knee towards you until you feel the stretch in your hip and glutes. Then hold.
- Repeat on the other side.

Make it easier:

- Instead of pulling from the back of your left leg, you can pull your right thigh toward you. It can be a little easier, especially if you have a hard time reaching behind your leg.

3. 90/90

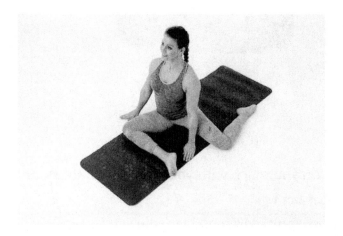

This stretch is also designed to give your hips more flexibility. Sitting all day can really tighten up these important joints. By making your hips more flexible, you may also reduce lower back pain.

It's called the 90/90 because you're basically making right angles with both your legs: one in front and one to the side. Then you'll switch so the front leg is to the side, and vice versa. Do this one sitting down on the floor.

- Sit down and bend your left leg in front of you so that your left ankle is pointing to the right and your left knee is bent at a right angle. Your left calf and knee should be on the ground. In this position, your hip is rotated outward.
- Now bend your right leg to the side so that your right knee has a right-angle bend and your foot is pointing right. Here your right hip is rotated internally, and your shin and ankle are on the ground. Make sure your right knee is in line with your hip.
- Hold, then switch so your right leg is in front and your left leg is to the side.

Again, you need to keep your back straight. You'll want to lean to one side, but avoid the temptation: keep both hips on the ground as much as you can.

Make it easier:

- Opening up the angle in your knees so it's not a complete right angle will make it a little easier to hold the pose.

4. Frog

The frog stretch is also great for opening up your hips (if you do yoga, this is also known as mandukasana). You might want to do this on a mat, because you start off on your hands and knees. If you're pregnant, make sure your tummy isn't pressing against the floor.

FROG STRETCH

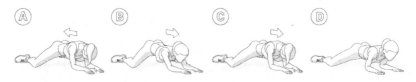

- Start on all fours, on your hands and knees in a tabletop position. Make sure your wrists are directly underneath your shoulders, not in front of them, and that your knees are directly under your hips. Keep your back flat and tummy tight, which will protect your back as well.
- Slowly slide both knees away from you: your left knee slides left, and your right knee slides right.

Allow them to slide until you can feel a nice stretch in your groin and inner thighs. Hold.

As you slide, rotate your ankles outward so the insides of your feet are against the floor.

You can go from being on your palms to resting on your elbows and forearms, and even your chest on the floor, as you become more flexible with this stretch.

It's important to come out of this stretch safely. If you go down to the forearms or chest, walk your hands back to tabletop. Return one hip at a time back to your starting position.

Make it easier:

- You may not be able to slide your knees wide at first. Slide until you feel the stretch, but don't push it too far.
- Put more weight on your hands, and gently rock back and forth until you can stretch.
- Try working on one hip at a time.

5. Butterfly

Yes, another hip opener! It's great for beginners if you find the previous two hard to get into. You also do this one sitting down, so it may be better than frog stretch for anyone with wrist issues. Make sure that you're not leaning to one side or the other.

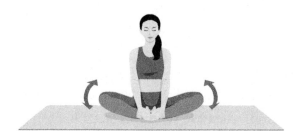

- Sit down with your legs bent in front of you and feet together, so your legs make a diamond shape.
- The closer your feet are to your groin, the deeper the stretch.
- You can lace your fingers under your pinky toes or hold your first two toes, or simply hold onto your ankles or shins.
- With each breath, settle a bit deeper into the stretch and hold.

If your hips are tight, your knees could be pretty high off the ground. Support them with blocks or cushions so that you can allow your thighs to fully relax.

Make it easier:

- If you have a hard time keeping your back straight, sit against a wall.
- You can also lie on your back and put your legs against the wall.
- Don't bring your feet in too close; let them relax a little farther away from your groin.

6. Calf

At the back of your lower legs, you'll find your calf muscles. They help you flex your feet, run, walk, jump, and stand up straight. The calf stretch is pretty simple.

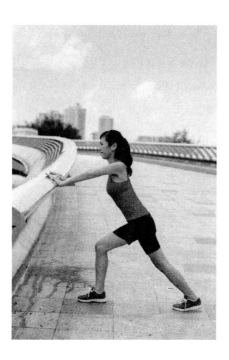

- Stand behind a chair and hold onto the top of it for balance.
- Step one foot back, making sure that the foot is flat on the ground.
- Bend your elbows, front knee, and hips forward until you feel the stretch, and hold.
- Repeat for the other leg.

Make it easier:

- Don't step back quite as far.

7. Standing lunge

While this will stretch out your hips, it also stretches out your whole leg: hamstrings, glutes, calves, and quadriceps, which are the muscles on the front of your thighs. You'll also practice maintaining your balance, which, as you know, is critical as you get older.

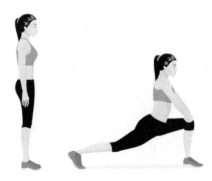

- Step your left leg back as comfortably as you can while bending your right knee. It's critical for your knee that you don't bend it too far forward; make sure it's in line with your right ankle. Keep your hips pointed forward and settle in the middle—don't lean to one side or the other.
- Rest your hands on your right thigh (not your knee!) for balance.
- Straighten your left leg without locking the knee. Tilt your pelvis forward to open up your hips (it's a small movement, but you'll feel it).
- Keep your tummy tight and back straight to protect your back as you hold the stretch.
- Switch.

Sometimes one hip wants to sag down to the floor, so keep them both in the same line.

Make it easier:

- If keeping your balance is an issue, do the stretch next to a chair that you can hold onto for balance instead of resting your hands on your thigh.
- Modify your knee bend so it's not 90 degrees.

Arm, neck, and back stretches

These stretches are not only important in keeping you flexible; they can make you feel better after a day sitting at the computer! As always, don't go into these cold. You can do arm circles or some other warmup to make sure your muscles are ready for the stretch.

Just as you probably found with lower body stretches that one side is more flexible than the other, you'll probably have the same difference in your upper body too. Again, don't give up on the weaker or less flexible side—give it the same attention as the other.

1. Overhead triceps stretch

Your triceps run up the back of your arm from the elbow to the shoulder. These muscles are very important for reaching up and lifting, so make sure they get a good stretch. You can either sit or stand with this one, so do whichever feels most comfortable.

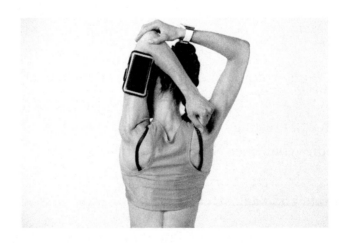

Reach your right arm straight up toward the ceiling, then bend your elbow so your hand is toward your back. Try to get that right hand as far as possible down your back to deepen the stretch.

- Put your left hand on top of your bent right elbow and gently push your arm and hand a little farther down your back. Hold.
- Switch.

Make it easier:

- You may not be flexible enough to get your hand down to the middle of your back. Let it go as far as you can, and then push (gently) with your left hand. You may only be able to reach the back of your neck, and that's okay.

2. Cross-body shoulder

Your shoulders are a pretty important part of your upper body and also help with lifting and reaching (and typing…). It's usually easiest to do this while you're standing.

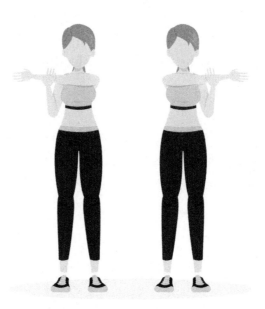

- Reach your right arm across your chest and hold it as straight as you can.
- Use your left hand to pull your right elbow in towards you as you keep the arm straight. The tighter your arm is to your chest, the deeper the stretch. Hold.
- Switch.

Make it easier:

- If your shoulders are tight, you won't be able to pull your arms too close. Pull until you feel the stretch, but don't go too far.

3. Standing bicep

These muscles run from your elbow to your wrist and are important for many types of movements, both in sports and at the office. You might find that if you do a lot of typing, your biceps get tight, so you will definitely feel this stretch.

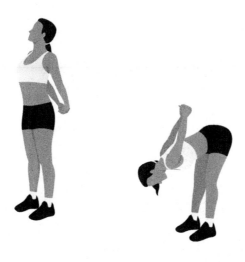

- While standing tall, push your arms behind you and lock your hands together.
- Slowly turn your hands so the palms are facing outward, and hold.

Make it easier:

- You can pull your hands farther apart or grip a towel between your hands. Just ensure the palms are facing outward.

4. Knee to chest

Although this stretch may at first seem like a lower body stretch, it actually benefits your lower back.

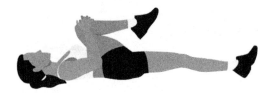

- Lie down on your back with your feet flat on the ground. Bend your right knee and hug it to your chest. Hold.

- Switch.

Make it easier:

- The closer you hug your knee, the deeper the stretch. You may not be able to pull it all the way to your chest at first.

5. Piriformis

If you haven't heard of this muscle, it helps rotate your hips and is one of your glutes. Stretching this muscle helps with back pain, especially with the sciatic nerve, which is why it's included in this section.

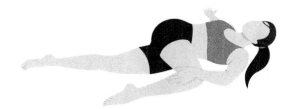

- Lie on your back with your feet flat on the ground.
- Bring your right knee up to your chest.
- With your left hand, pull your knee towards your left shoulder. Hold.
- Switch.

Make it easier:

- If you're not very flexible (yet), you may not be able to pull your knee very high. That's okay, just stretch as far as you can.

6. Lumbar flexion

This is just another phrase for bending forward. Many Americans with tight muscles in their back and hips have a hard time doing this, so don't feel bad if you need to work your way up. The better your lumbar flexion, the less back pain you'll experience.

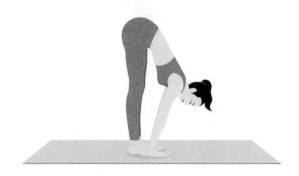

There's a progression for this stretch depending on how flexible you are at the moment. If you can't keep your legs straight while bending forward at the hips and touching your toes, start with one of the easier stretches and work your way up.

- Supine

Lie on your back with your knees bent. Bring both knees up to your chest and grab with your hands, tugging until you feel the stretch. Hold. (It may feel better if you rock gently back and forth while holding your knees.)

- Seated

Sit in a chair and bend forward from your hips, as far as you can go. Hold. You can increase the stretch by holding onto your ankles.

- Standing

While standing, bend forward from your hips as far as you can. (This can also stretch your hamstrings.)

Make it easier:

- Go back a stretch. If you can't do seated, then start with supine, for instance.

7. Seated spinal twist

You'll be able to stretch your spine and sides with this twist.
Keep your hips even and don't let yourself sink to one side.

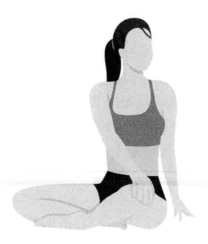

- Sit with your legs straight out in front of you.
- Bend your right knee, then bring your right leg
  across your body and rest your right foot next to the
  outside of your left thigh. You'll probably feel a bit of
  a stretch here, but there's more.
- Stretch your right arm behind you so that you're
  resting on your fingertips, which will twist your
  body to the right.

- Reach your left arm to your right knee and cradle it, pulling your leg a bit to the left while your spine is twisted to the right. Hold.
- Switch.

Make it easier:

- You may not be able to twist so much to the right.
- Some people find it easier to put their left elbow against the inside of their right knee and push gently (instead of pulling with the arm).

  8. Neck stretch

Be very gentle and slow any time you're stretching your neck. Don't twist or jerk it suddenly. You can stand or sit for these stretches.

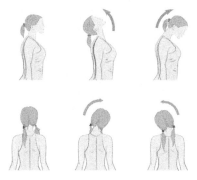

- With your back held straight and your head directly over your neck, slowly drop your chin to your chest and hold.
- Return to center, then drop your head back so your chin is in the air. Hold.
- Return to center. Turn your head slowly to the right as far as you can, and hold.
- Return to center. Turn to the left and hold.

Yoga poses

Some of the stretches listed above are also yoga poses; for example, the frog stretch for your hips is also a yoga pose. You'll find a few more poses that are suitable for beginners and also give you a nice stretch.

It's sometimes helpful when doing yoga poses to pace your breath so that you do one movement on the inhale and another on the exhale. Breathe as you're holding these poses as well. Many of them stretch a variety of muscles in your body.

1. Easy pose/sukhsana

Great for tight hips, and very simple.

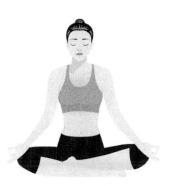

- Sit up straight on a mat and cross your legs at the shins.
- Tuck each foot under the opposite knee. Notice which leg goes on top.
- Put your hands on your knees, palms down. Make sure that you're sitting tall, with hips even and relax your feet and thighs, then hold.
- Switch so that the bottom leg is on top.

Make it easier:

- If your hips are tight, don't sit on the floor. Prop your butt up with some cushions so your hips are higher than your knees and ankles.

- If your hips are super tight, do this in a chair and cross one leg at a time.

2. Child's pose (balasana)

This one helps you stretch out your back and hips.

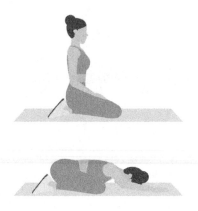

- Kneel so that you're sitting on your knees, butt on your heels.
- Lean forward with your butt still on your heels and rest your forehead on the floor.
- Stretch your arms back alongside your legs with the palm facing up. Hold.

Make it easier:

- It's hard for a lot of people to put their foreheads on the floor. Instead, when you lean forward, put your forearms on the floor and rest your forehead on that.

3. Tree (vrksansana)

This is an excellent stretch for working on your balance and is great for your legs and core. You'll be on one leg, so start off next to a chair or something you can grab hold of if you start to wobble! The secret to keeping your balance is to look at something that doesn't move, like a spot on the floor or artwork on the wall.

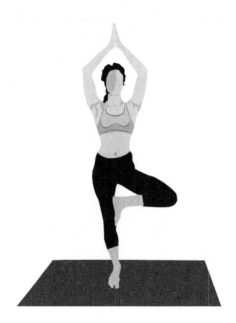

- Stand straight up with your weight equally balanced on both feet.
- Lift your right leg and bend the knee. Keep your left leg straight but knees soft, not locked.

- Place your right foot flat on the inside of your left thigh. The higher the foot, the deeper the stretch.
- Keep your hips straight and in line with each other. Press your foot and inner thigh against each other to make sure one hip doesn't pop out of line, and hold.
- Switch.

Make it easier:

- Start with your right foot against your left ankle or calf and move your foot up as you become more flexible and can maintain your balance.

4. Downward-facing dog (adho muka svasana)

This is a key pose for many yoga sequences and can help you lengthen your body and improve flexibility in a multitude of areas. Many beginners are not able to do this with straight legs, so if you need to bend them go for it.

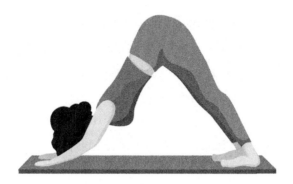

Keep your hands shoulder-width apart and your feet hip-width apart, no narrower. Keep your back straight.

- Start on all fours on your hand and knees, with your toes tucked in and your wrists directly under your shoulders.
- Exhale to push your hips back and up, which will straighten your legs (eventually).
- Engage your arms, but make sure your shoulders stay down and don't start creeping up toward your ears.
- Pull your tummy in.
- Press through your heels and hold—you can pedal your feet up and down if that feels good to you.

Make it easier:

- Use blocks underneath your hands or rolled-up mats under your heels to reduce the stretch.
- Especially if your wrists are bugging you, come down onto your forearms.

5. Bridge (Setu Bandha Sarvangasana)

Looking for a great back stretch? It's a beginner's back bend that will also help out your core.

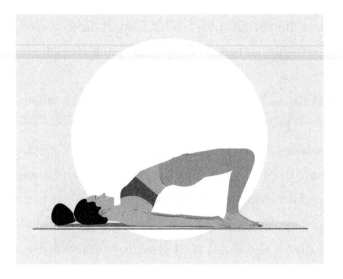

- Lie on your back with your feet flat on the ground with your knees bent and hip-width apart.
- Move your feet closer to your butt, raising your hips as you go.

- Reach your arms underneath and lace your hands together.
- Press down through your heels and lift your thighs as high as you can. Hold.

Make it easier:

- Hold a towel in your hands if you can't clasp your hands.
- Squeeze a block or towel between your thighs as you lift.

6. Warrior II (virabhadrasana II)

You'll get a nice hip stretch with this pose.

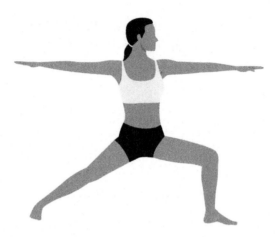

- Stand with a wide stance and stretch your arms out so your ankles are under your wrists.
- Turn your right foot and your right knee out to the right.
- Bend your right knee so it's over your right ankle, and make sure your weight is still even between your two feet.
- Engage your arms and turn your head to the right. Hold.
- Straighten both your legs and return to the wide stance, then switch sides.

Make it easier:

- Perform this pose against a wall with a block or towel between your thigh and the wall. Push against the wall. This will help with balance but also make sure your knee doesn't start to wobble towards the front.

7. Extended Triangle (utthita trikonasana)

This pose provides a whole-body stretch.

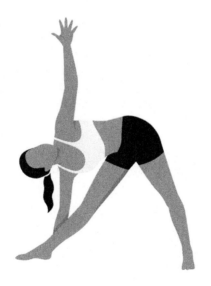

- Stand with your feet 3–4 feet apart.
- Turn your left foot in a little bit and your right foot out. Make sure your heels are still in line with each other.
- Exhale and stretch to the right from your hips, ensuring that you're still in line with your right hip and that your left hip is firmly in position.
- When you're as far as possible, reach your right hand (palm forward) to the ground and your left arm straight up overhead. Your shoulders, arms, and hands should form a straight line at a right angle to the floor.
- Rest your hand against your shin, calf, knee, or the ground - however far you can reach without losing your form. Hold.
- Switch.

Make it easier:

- Use a long block to rest your hand on so that you can keep your back straight without rounding it, or otherwise falling into bad form.

8. Upward-facing dog (urdhva mukha svansana)

If you're looking for a deep back and core stretch, this pose is for you. It's a back bend that will also help you stretch your wrists.

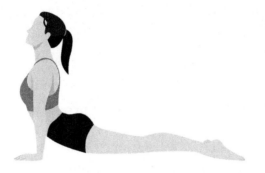

- Lie down on your belly and rest your hands on either side of your tummy, with your fingers pointing forward.
- Inhale and lift your head and chest, pushing off the ground. Straighten your arms completely without locking your elbows.
- Lift your knees, pelvis, and legs up off the ground while keeping the tops of your feet on the ground.
- Roll your shoulders so they're down and back. Hold.

Make it easier:

- Do cobra pose instead: leave your legs and feet on the floor and your hands under your shoulder blades, then lift your upper body.
- Use blocks at your sides for your hands.

Put it all together: 14-day stretch program

Ready to put together a program? Here's a sample one that you can use for the two-week reset program. You can also add in a yoga pose or two, depending on how your body feels that day.

Day 1 - four stretches

- Standing hamstring
- Calf
- Cross-body shoulder
- Lumbar flexion

Day 2 - none

Day 3 - five stretches

- Figure 4
- Butterfly
- Overhead triceps
- Knee to chest
- Neck

Day 4 - none

Day 5 - six stretches

- 90/90
- Frog
- Standing lunge
- Standing bicep
- Piriformis
- Seated spinal twist

Day 6 - none

Day 7 - all stretches

Day 8 - none

Day 9 - all stretches

Day 10 - none

Day 11 - all stretches

Day 12 - all stretches

Day 13 - all stretches

Day 14 - all stretches

Inspiration: Malaika Arora Khan

She's an Indian actress and TV personality well known for her Instagram posts. She is a big devotee of clean eating.

Even with her busy schedule, she rarely eats out, preferring instead to stay home and make her own delicious food.

She also practices intermittent fasting, so that she eats during a specific window of time during the day. This gives the body time to rest after digestion, and many celebrities swear by it.

Food for thought

Time to look at how often (or not) you currently stretch and how you can work the 14-day program.

- Do you spend time stretching now?
- Are you familiar with any of the stretches mentioned in the chapter so that you can easily work them into your routine?
- What are your least flexible areas, and which stretches will you incorporate specifically for them?
- What time during the day will you focus on your stretching, including the light warmup, so you don't go in cold?

Chapter Summary

You've got a simple 14-day plan to follow for stretching, and you can start exactly where you are now. Make the modifications if you need to so you don't get hurt—after all, no one has to watch you doing these!

6

TIME TO DANCE!

"The purpose of training is to tighten up the slack, toughen the body, and polish the spirit."

— MORIHEI USHIBA

Your specific strategy for dance will depend on the type of dancing you're planning to do and how familiar you are with it. If it's something you've done before (but haven't done in a while), don't expect muscle memory to kick in right away. Start at the beginner level until things come back to you.

Your fitness level is probably different from what it was back then too, so don't expect your body to be able to do the same things or at the same level of intensity. Just like with stretching, start where you are. If you stopped dancing 20 years ago, just accept that you're a beginner again and look forward to learning new things. You may be able to dance in a way that you couldn't when you were younger.

How much dancing do you need?

The current recommendations for aerobic activity, the kind that gets your heart pumping, differ according to how hard you go at it. For moderate intensity, you need 150 hours a week, which is 2½ hours a day. If you're going harder with vigorous intensity, you need only one hour and 15 minutes a day.[1]

What a lot of people don't recognize is that you don't have to do all that activity at once. In fact, it's better if you don't. If you prefer a dance style that's fast-paced and gets your heart pumping, it's better to do that for 25 minutes three times a week than to do one class on the weekends for 75 minutes.

And it's the same with moderate activity too. Don't break a sweat for an hour and 15 minutes twice a week; it's better to divvy up your 150 minutes for 30 minutes, five days a week.

The trick with aerobic activity is that doing some is better than doing none. Many people think if they can't fit in an hour-long workout that they should just skip the whole thing instead. Don't be one of those people! You might not be able to get 30 continuous minutes of exercise on some days, but you can do 10 minutes in the morning, 10 minutes at lunch, and 10 minutes before dinner.

A little bit of exercise is so much better than none, though you should shoot for the targets mentioned as the minimum. You can absolutely do more as you get stronger and start shedding weight. You just have to start somewhere, and if you haven't been exercising at all, build your routine.

Your next question might be, what's the difference between moderate and vigorous intensity? In terms of walking, moderate activity is a brisk walk (not a slow amble at the mall where you're checking out the store displays). Vigorous is running or jogging.

It varies from person to person, but in general, moderate movement feels somewhat hard. It's not a walk in the park, because you are breathing harder, but you're not out of breath. You'll start to sweat about 10 minutes in, and while you can talk with a friend, you don't have enough breath to sing.

If you're not sweating and it doesn't feel hard and your breathing hasn't changed, it doesn't count as moderate. You need to pick up the pace or make the activity harder in some way. For example, if you were out walking, you could decide to climb a hill, and that would get you in the zone.

In contrast, vigorous activity feels hard. You can't talk without needing a breath, you're sweating pretty soon into the movement, and your breath is coming fast and hard. If you were walking briskly (moderate) and wanted to make it vigorous, you could start climbing a very steep hill.

What types of dance are good for aerobic activity?

Not all dance routines get your pulse pounding. For example, many ballet classes, while technically difficult, don't count as aerobic unless you're skilled enough to be doing a lot of leaping and fast-paced movements.

The music may also influence how vigorously you're dancing because an upbeat tempo can really get your heart pumping! You may find that you prefer certain dance styles (or prefer to avoid them) due to the kind of music that accompanies them.

1. Moderate dancing

- Ballroom, swing

These types of dances are done with partners. If you have a partner, you can go to a dance studio, though some allow dancers without partners and you'll get paired up when you get there.

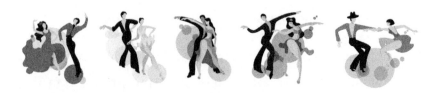

Ballroom is often set to waltz or tango music. Swing dancing developed with jazz in the early 20th century and is often associated with big band ensembles. Dancers might flip, spin, and lift their partners during the course of the dance.

- Square

This is also a partnered type of folk dance that usually includes four couples. They form a square facing each other, and a caller announces the steps to perform.

- Jazz

Also developed in the 20th century, jazz is much influenced by jazz music (as you might have guessed) and includes modern dance steps as well. A lot of Broadway and Hollywood choreography is based on jazz dance. Many pro jazz dancers start off with ballet.

- Line

As you might guess from the name, the dancers form lines and do choreograph steps on repeat. Country music is a popular choice for line dancing, but you can line dance to all kinds of music.

- Tap

For this type of dance, you'll have tap shoes with metal plates typically on the toes and heels so that you make different sounds while dancing different steps. It's similar to Irish clogging. A lot of the choreography can be improvised, so it's often linked to jazz music, though anything rhythmic with a beat will work.

2. Vigorous dancing

- Zumba

Technically this isn't a dance style, but an aerobics class that incorporates dance movements. It's usually fast and upbeat, so you can definitely get a good workout in.

- Hip-hop

This style is based on street dancing and goes with hip-hop music. It may involve choreography or can be mostly improvised. In addition to steps like the humpty, the cabbage patch, and the running man, there are a lot of body movements like krumping or popping and locking. They're very high energy, and the footwork tends to be complicated.

- Salsa

This Latin dance is typically done partnered, and it can be very high energy. It originally came from Cuba and is relatively easy to learn.

14-day program

How much you'll dance depends on whether you've chosen a moderate or a vigorous style. However, if you haven't been exercising in a while, check with your doctor first and start off a little more slowly. If half an hour of dancing is a little too much for you right now, that's okay. Start with 10–15 minutes of the dance you want to try and work your way up.

Don't be afraid to change it up, either. Maybe one day you have a partner and want to do some salsa, and another day you're more in the mood for hip-hop. In the schedule, we've focused mainly on 25 to 30 minutes, but do 10–15 instead if that's too much.

- Day 1 - 10 minutes of dance as warmup
- Day 2 - 20 minutes
- Day 3 - none
- Day 4 - 20 minutes
- Day 5 - none
- Day 6 - 25 minutes
- Day 7 - none
- Day 8 - 25–30 minutes
- Day 9 - none

- Day 10 - 25–30 minutes
- Day 11 - none
- Day 12 - 25–30 minutes
- Day 13 - none
- Day 14 - 25–30 minutes

Inspiration: Kayla Itsines

She's a well-known trainer in Australia and the co-founder of a huge fitness community called Sweat. In addition to all the workouts she does, Kayla is known for her clean eating regimen. She loves to eat as many whole foods as possible.

Food for thought

As with stretching, it's a good idea to look at where you are with dance now and how and when you can fit it into your schedule.

- Are you dancing right now?
- If not, are you doing moderate or vigorous exercise as recommended during the week?
- What kind of dance would you like to try, and will you go to a studio or watch videos?
- How will you arrange your day so that you get your 25–30 minutes in?

Chapter Summary

Dancing is a fun way to get your heart pumping, and you can do a little bit each day so you don't injure yourself. Pick something fun and interesting with music that you like and go for it.

---

1. https://www.cdc.gov/physicalactivity/basics/adults/index.htm

7

YOUR 14-DAY MEAL PLAN (WITH SHOPPING LIST!)

"Today I will do what others won't, so tomorrow I can accomplish what others can't."

— JERRY RICE

A s you've learned, exercise alone won't help you lose weight. You've also got to feed your body clean energy. The clean eating plan described earlier will do much more than "just" help you lose weight: you'll experience less inflammation, better moods, better skin, and a host of other benefits, including less brain fog.

Your 14-day plan overview

All the recipes and ideas that follow are based on the clean eating principles you learned about earlier in the book. Remember to drink plenty of water on the plan. This is designed for you to change your relationship to food and lead a healthier lifestyle; it isn't a "diet" that you go off when you're feeling deprived or because you lost the weight you wanted to lose.

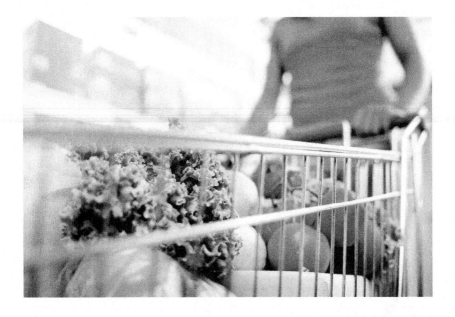

This 14-day plan will be the basis of your nutrition past the 14 days of your reset. You'll be eating breakfast, lunch, dinner, and a snack each day, so you won't feel deprived. Breakfast is based on detox smoothies, which you can continue after the two weeks, or find a few other clean breakfasts that work for you.

Day 1

- Detox smoothie breakfast: Easy Detox Smoothie
- Lunch: Quick Taco Salad in a Jar
- Snack: Apple slices with almond butter
- Dinner: Southwestern Sweet Potato and Egg Hash

Day 2

- Detox smoothie breakfast: Green Protein Smoothie
- Lunch: Cold Pasta Salad
- Snack: Fresh veggies with guacamole
- Dinner: Tahini Chicken with Kale and Squash

Day 3

- Detox smoothie breakfast: Peaches and Cream Oatmeal Smoothie
- Lunch: Spicy Chili with Fire-Roasted Tomatoes (slow cooker)
- Snack: Sweet Potato Toast
- Dinner: Pan-seared Shrimp with Rosemary Zoodles

Day 4

- Detox smoothie breakfast: Vegan Cucumber Smoothie

- Lunch: Veggie Panini with Roasted Peppers and Goat Cheese
- Snack: Coconut Brownie Energy Balls
- Dinner: Vegan Spaghetti Squash with Mushroom Marinara

Day 5

- Detox smoothie breakfast: Mango Smoothie
- Lunch: Soba Salad with Honey-Ginger dressing
- Snack: Apple slices with almond butter
- Dinner: Sheet-Pan Chicken with Rainbow Veggies

Day 6

- Detox smoothie breakfast: Green Protein Smoothie
- Lunch: Quick Taco Salad in a Jar
- Snack: Small handful mixed nuts
- Dinner: Pad See Ew With Zoodles

Day 7

- Detox smoothie breakfast: Vegan Cucumber Smoothie
- Lunch: Greek Goddess Chicken Wraps
- Snack: Fresh veggies with guacamole
- Dinner: Southwestern Sweet Potato and Egg Hash

Day 8

- Detox smoothie breakfast: Easy Detox Smoothie
- Lunch: Greek Yogurt Egg Salad Sandwich
- Snack: Ham & Cheese Apple Wraps
- Dinner: Winter Veggie Gratin

Day 9

- Detox smoothie breakfast: Green Protein Smoothie
- Lunch: Grown-Up Grilled Cheese Sandwich
- Snack: Coconut Brownie Energy Balls
- Dinner: Taco Skillet

Day 10

- Detox smoothie breakfast: Mango Smoothie
- Lunch: Cold Pasta Salad
- Snack: Apple slices with almond butter
- Dinner: Sheet-Pan Chicken with Rainbow Veggies

Day 11

- Detox smoothie breakfast: Peaches and Cream Oatmeal Smoothie
- Lunch: Soba Salad with Honey-Ginger dressing
- Snack: Ham & Cheese Apple Wraps

- Dinner: Vegan Spaghetti Squash with Mushroom Marinara

Day 12

- Detox smoothie breakfast: Mango Smoothie
- Lunch: Quick Taco Salad in a Jar
- Snack: Sweet Potato Toast
- Dinner: Tahini Chicken with Kale and Squash

Day 13

- Detox smoothie breakfast: Easy Detox Smoothie
- Lunch: Spicy Chili with Fire-Roasted Tomatoes (slow cooker)
- Snack: Fresh veggies with guacamole
- Dinner: Winter Veggie Gratin

Day 14

- Detox smoothie breakfast: Peaches and Cream Oatmeal Smoothie
- Lunch: Veggie Panini with Roasted Peppers and Goat Cheese
- Snack: Small handful of mixed nuts
- Dinner: Pan-seared Shrimp with Rosemary Zoodles

The recipes

- Detox smoothies

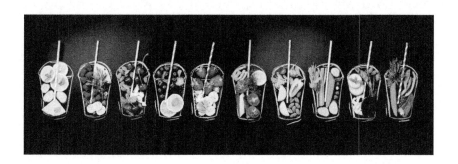

1. Easy Detox Smoothie

- ½ cup water or orange juice
- 1 green apple
- ½ cup frozen pineapple
- ½ frozen banana
- 1 cup (fresh) spinach
- ½ inch peeled and minced ginger
- 1 small handful cilantro (skip if it tastes soapy to you)
- 1 tablespoon fresh lime juice.

Blend until smooth, then pour and serve right away.

2. Green Protein Smoothie

- ½ cup unsweetened almond milk
- 1 tbsp. almond butter

- 1 banana
- 2 cups fresh baby spinach

Blend until smooth, adding water if you want a more liquid consistency.

3. Peaches and Cream Oatmeal Smoothie

- 1 cup frozen peaches
- 1 cup each baby spinach, Greek yogurt, and almond milk
- ¼ cup oatmeal
- ¼ tsp vanilla extract

Blend until smooth.

4. Mango Smoothie

- ⅓ avocado
- 1 cup spinach
- ½ cup each mango, blueberries, almond milk (or soy milk), and ice cubes
- ½ a lime, squeezed

Blend until smooth.

5. Vegan Cucumber Smoothie

- 1½ cup water
- 1 cup pineapple
- 1 cucumber
- 12 dates
- 1 lemon, squeezed

Blend until smooth.

- Lunches

Your lunches don't have to be time-consuming. Some can be prepared in 10 minutes or less.

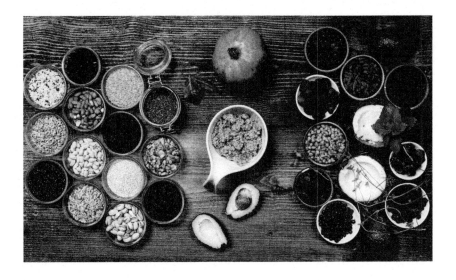

1. Taco Salad in a Jar

Serves 6.

- ½ pound ground turkey
- 1 tsp chili powder
- ½ tsp cumin
- ¼ tsp garlic powder
- ¼ tsp salt
- ½ cup each broken whole-grain tortilla chips, salsa, and reduced fat shredded cheddar
- 3 cups chopped romaine lettuce
- 1 cup halved cherry tomatoes

For the dressing:

- 2 tbsp Greek yogurt
- 2 tbsp avocado
- ¼ cup salsa
- Juice of 1 lime

For the salad: Heat skillet over medium heat and add ground turkey. Heat until cooked through, then stir in chili powder, cumin, garlic powder, and salt. Place in a bowl to cool.

Meanwhile, divide broken tortilla chips between the six jars. Layer with salsa, shredded cheddar, romaine, turkey mixture, and cherry tomatoes.

If you like, for the dressing, blend together yogurt, avocado, salsa, and lime.

Top the jars with the dressing and seal. Best kept in the fridge for 1–2 days.

2. Cold Pasta Salad

Serves 4.

- 6 oz. pasta
- Olive oil for drizzling
- 1 tbsp pine nuts
- 12 big fresh basil leaves
- 2 tbsp grated Parmesan
- 1 clove garlic
- ¼ tsp salt
- 1 cup halved cherry tomatoes
- ⅛ cup olive oil
- ½ cup fresh chopped and drained mozzarella

Boil a pot of water over high heat and cook pasta according to package directions. When done, drain and rinse with cold water, then place in bowl with drizzle of olive oil to keep from sticking.

With an immersion blender, combine pine nuts, basil leaves, Parmesan, garlic, and salt for pesto. Add in ⅛ cup olive oil as you blend.

In a bowl, mix pasta, pesto, cherry tomatoes and mozzarella.

3. Spicy Chili with Fire-Roasted Tomatoes (slow cooker)

Serves 6.

- 1 lb. lean ground beef
- 1 diced yellow onion
- 2 minced garlic cloves
- 15 oz. rinsed and drained organic kidney beans
- 15 oz. rinsed and drained organic black beans
- 14½ oz. can fire-roasted tomatoes
- 6 oz canned tomato paste
- 2 tbsp. chili powder
- ½ tsp black pepper
- ½ tsp red pepper or to taste
- 1½ cup water
- Salt to taste

Heat large skillet over medium heat and add ground beef, onion, and garlic. Cook until beef is no longer pink and drain off fat.

Add contents to slow cooker along with beans, tomatoes, tomato paste, chili powder, black pepper, red pepper, 1½ cup water, and salt to taste.

Cover and cook on low setting for 6–8 hours until ready to serve.

4. Veggie Panini with Roasted Peppers and Goat Cheese

Serves 4.

- 1 cup roasted peppers
- 8 slices whole grain bread
- 4 sweet onion slices
- 4 tomato slices
- 4 tbsp goat cheese
- 1 tbsp fresh thyme
- Salt and pepper to taste

Slice roasted peppers into strips. Brush oil over one side of eight slices of bread and heat the panini press (or nonstick skillet) to medium heat or 350 degrees. To the dry side of four slices of bread, add peppers, sweet onion, tomato, goat cheese, thyme, and salt and pepper to taste. Top with the dry side of remaining four slices and press sandwich until hot and crispy.

5. Soba Salad with Honey-Ginger dressing

Serves 6.

For dressing:

- 4 tbsp. light soy sauce (tamari)
- 2 tbsp rice wine vinegar
- 1 tbsp honey

- 2 tbsp sesame oil
- 2-inch peeled and sliced ginger

For salad:

- 2 carrots
- 1 cucumber
- 1 endive
- 7 oz soba (buckwheat) noodles
- 1 tbsp toasted sesame seeds
- 2 tbsp chopped chives
- 1 tbsp pine nuts (optional)

In a small bowl, whisk together soy sauce (tamari), vinegar, honey, sesame oil, and ginger.

Peel and slice carrots, cucumber, and endive to a uniform size and shape.

Boil water over high heat and add noodles per package directions, then drain and rinse with cold water. Toss in a bowl with the dressing. Add the peeled veggies, sesame seeds, chives, and pine nuts if desired. Eat hot or cold.

6. Greek Goddess Chicken Wraps

Serves 4.

For chicken marinade:

- 2 tbsp olive oil
- 1 lb. sliced boneless skinless chicken breast
- 2 minced or grated garlic cloves
- 1 tbsp smoked paprika
- ¼ cup fresh oregano
- 1 sliced lemon
- Salt and pepper to taste

For the dressing:

- ¼ cup water
- ½ cup roasted pistachios
- 2 tbsp lemon juice
- 1 clove garlic
- 1 cup fresh basil
- 1 jalapeno (optional)
- Salt to taste

For fries:

- 2 potatoes cut into matchsticks
- 2 tbsp olive oil
- Salt and pepper to taste

For pita sandwiches:

- 4 pita bread (if desired)
- 1 head butter lettuce
- 2 Persian cucumbers cut into matchsticks
- 1 sliced avocado
- ⅓ cup pitted kalamata olives

The day before, place olive oil, chicken, garlic, smoked paprika, oregano, lemon, and salt and pepper into a ziplock bag and shake to coat. Marinate in the fridge.

For the dressing, blend water, roasted pistachios, lemon juice, garlic, basil, jalapeno (optional), and salt. Add more water if you want to thin it out.

Preheat oven to 425 degrees. Put chicken in a 9x13 inch baking dish and roast for 20–25 minutes or until cooked through.

Meanwhile, toss two potatoes with olive oil and salt and pepper to taste. Bake them for 20–25 minutes, tossing halfway through.

Stuff pitas (if using) with butter lettuce and add fries and chicken. On top, add Persian cucumbers, avocado, and olives. Drizzle dressing over each one.

7. Greek Yogurt Egg Salad Sandwich

Serves 4.

- 1 baguette cut into 4 servings
- 8 hard-boiled eggs
- ⅔ cup Greek yogurt
- 1 tbsp mayonnaise
- 1 tsp dill
- Salt and pepper to taste

For toppings:

- 2 cup arugula
- 2 sliced tomatoes
- 1 sliced avocado

Peel and slice eight cold boiled eggs. Mash with Greek yogurt, mayonnaise, dill, and salt and pepper.

Pile in toasted baguette and top with arugula, tomatoes, and avocado.

8. Grown-Up Grilled Cheese Sandwich

Serves 1.

- 2 slices bread
- Olive oil

- Tomatoes (to taste), sliced
- 6 fresh large basil leaves
- Salt and pepper to taste
- 2 oz. mozzarella

Preheat oven to 350 degrees. Brush one side of bread with olive oil. On dry side, add tomato slices, basil leaves, salt and pepper, and mozzarella.

Pop sandwich in oven between 2 cookie sheets (you can add a little weight to the top) and bake for about 20 minutes or until your cheese is melted. If you like, sprinkle a little balsamic vinegar on top and dig in.

- Snacks

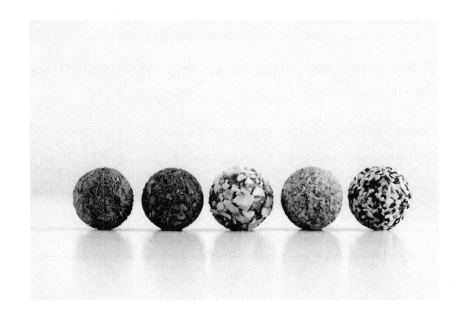

1. Coconut Brownie Energy Balls

24–30 balls (1 ball/serving)

- 1 cup raisins
- ⅓ cup shredded coconut
- 1 cup cashews
- ¼ cup cocoa powder
- 1 tsp vanilla extract
- ¼ tsp salt
- Pinch of cinnamon

Soak raisins in hot water. Let soften for five minutes, then drain.

Put shredded coconut on a plate for rolling and set aside.

Add softened raisins, cashews, cocoa powder, vanilla extract, salt, and cinnamon to a food processor. Pulse until it has the texture of sand.

Roll the dough into little balls and then roll on coconut plate. Let chill for 30 minutes. They'll keep up to a week in the fridge in an airtight container.

2. Sweet Potato Toast

Serves 4.

- 2 sweet potatoes, sliced into about 4 slices per tater
- Almond butter or guacamole

Toast spuds in toaster oven or in toaster (2 cycles). Once cooked, spread with topping: almond butter or guacamole.

3. Ham & Cheese Apple Wraps

Serves 2.

- 1 apple, your choice
- 8 slices deli ham
- 8 slices cheddar or Colby Jack cheese

Slice apple of your choice into eight wedges.

Place ham on plate and fold each slice in half. Add a cheese slice to each ham fold, then use to wrap up each apple wedge.

- Dinners

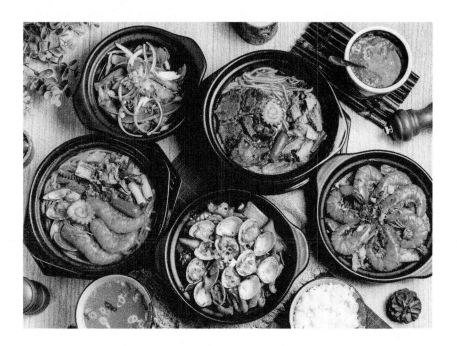

1. Southwestern Sweet Potato and Egg Hash

Serves 1.

- ¾ cup peeled and diced sweet potatoes
- 2 tsp water
- 1 tsp plus ¼ tsp olive oil
- ⅔ cup chopped red bell pepper
- ¼ tsp chili powder
- ⅛ tsp salt
- ⅛ tsp ground cumin
- ¼ cup canned black beans

- 1 egg

Microwave sweet potatoes on high with water for about four minutes and let stand for 5.

Heat 1 tsp olive oil in skillet over medium-high heat and add potatoes, pepper, chili powder, salt, and cumin. Cook until potatoes are crispy. Add black beans and then place on a plate.

Reduce the heat to medium and add ¼ tsp olive oil to the skillet. Crack one egg in and cook until whites are set, then place egg on tomato mixture. Top with salsa or dressing of your choice.

2. Pan-seared Shrimp with Rosemary Zoodles

Serves 1.

- 2 tsp olive oil
- 6 oz deveined shrimp
- ¼ cup thinly sliced red onion
- ½ tsp minced garlic
- 1½ cup zoodles (zucchini spiralized into noodles)
- 5 halved cherry tomatoes
- 1 tsp. fresh lemon juice
- ¼ tsp chopped fresh rosemary
- Salt to taste

Heat 1 tsp olive oil in a skillet over medium-high heat. Cook shrimp about two minutes on each side. Remove from the pan and keep warm.

Keep pan at medium-high and add 1 tsp olive oil, swirling to coat. Saute red onion and minced garlic until onions are tender, about four minutes.

Add zoodles, cherry tomatoes, fresh lemon juice, rosemary, and salt. Cook until warmed through and top with shrimp.

3. Tahini Chicken with Kale and Squash

Serves 1.

For dressing:

- 2½ tbsp fresh lemon juice
- 1 garlic clove
- ¼ cup tahini
- 1 to 3 tbsp cold water

For chicken and veggies:

- 1 tsp olive oil
- 3 oz cubed boneless skinless chicken thigh
- 1 clove plus ½ tsp finely chopped garlic
- ⅛ tsp plus ⅛ tsp salt
- ½ c. cubed butternut squash
- ½ tsp finely chopped peeled ginger

- ⅛ tsp black pepper
- ½ cup chicken stock
- ½ cup chopped kale
- ⅓ cup cooked whole grain rice

To make dressing, process lemon juice and garlic in food processor until garlic is roughly chopped. Add tahini and pulse 10 seconds or so. Add cold water 1 tbsp at a time until it's thin enough to drizzle.

Add olive oil to pan warmed over medium-high heat and swirl to coat. Cook chicken sprinkled with ⅛ tsp salt for 5 minutes or until browned—don't stir.

Add butternut squash, garlic, ginger, black pepper, and ⅛ tsp salt. Cook, stirring frequently, about one minute.

Add in chicken stock and bring to simmer. Reduce heat to medium-low and cover. Cook until squash is tender, about 15 minutes. Add kale and cover; cook about one more minute (kale starts to wilt if it's done for longer). Pour over 1½ tbsp dressing and serve on rice.

4. Vegan Spaghetti Squash with Mushroom Marinara

Serves 4.

- 1 spaghetti squash
- 4 tbsp olive oil
- Salt and pepper

- 1 carton (1 pint) sliced cremini mushrooms
- 2 cloves minced garlic
- 1 tbsp chopped thyme
- 2 tsp rosemary
- 2 cups marinara sauce
- 4 tbsp nutritional yeast

Prepare squash: Preheat oven to 400 degrees. Cut in half and remove seeds; brush with 1 tbsp olive oil. Salt and pepper to taste; place cut side down on parchment-lined baking sheet and roast for 35–40 minutes or until it cuts easily with a fork.

Heat 3 tbsp olive oil in a skillet over medium heat. Add mushrooms and cook for five minutes. Add garlic and sauté about one minute, then stir in thyme and rosemary. Season with salt and pepper and remove to a plate.

Turn heat down to medium-low and heat marinara sauce until warm, about five minutes.

Take the squash out of the oven and shred it with a fork. Divide into four servings and top with marinara, veggies, and 1 tbsp nutritional yeast per serving.

5. Sheet-Pan Chicken with Rainbow Veggies

Serves 4.

For sauce:

- 1 tbsp sesame oil
- 2 tbsp honey
- 2 tbsp soy sauce (tamari)

For chicken and veggies:

- 1 lb. boneless skinless chicken breasts
- 2 diced red bell peppers
- 2 diced yellow bell peppers
- 3 sliced carrots
- ½ head of broccoli cut into florets
- 2 diced red onions
- 2 tbsp olive oil
- Salt and pepper

Preheat oven to 400 degrees. Whisk sesame oil, honey, and soy sauce (tamari) together. Brush evenly over chicken.

On the sheet pan, arrange bell peppers, carrots, broccoli, and red onions. Toss to coat with olive oil and season to taste.

Put the chicken on the tray and roast until the chicken is done, about 20–25 minutes.

6. Pad See Ew With Zoodles

Serves 2.

For steak marinade:

- 5 oz flank steak cut into bite-size slices about ⅛ of an inch thick
- ½ tsp salt
- ½ tsp plus 2 tbsp tamari
- 1 tsp avocado oil
- 1 tsp coconut sugar

For veggies and other parts of meal:

- 2 zucchinis
- ⅓ cup raw cashews
- 1 tbsp plus 2 tsp avocado oil
- 1 tbsp minced, peeled ginger
- 3 minced garlic cloves
- 2 tbsp tamari
- 1 small bunch chopped bok choy separated into leaves and stems
- 2 tsp rice vinegar
- 1 egg

Prepare steak ahead of time by placing steak, salt, ½ tsp tamari, 1 tsp avocado oil, and coconut sugar in a zip-top bag.

Shake to coat steak, and marinate at least 20 minutes up to overnight.

Spiralize your zucchinis into noodles and let stand about 10 minutes over a strainer to drain.

Heat skillet to medium and dry toast cashews, then remove from pan. Return to medium-high heat and add 1 tbsp avocado oil. When it shimmers, add ginger; garlic; bok choy stems; 2 tbsp tamari, and 2 tbsp water. Cook about four minutes or until bok choy is tender-crisp. Add bok choy leaves and rice vinegar to cook until leaves wilt, 1–2 minutes. Push everything to the side and crack in an egg; cook until set and then toss with veggies to combine. Remove them to plate.

Wipe out the pan, bring back to medium-high, and add 2 tsp avocado oil. When it shimmers, add in the marinated flank steak, shaking off excess before you put the steak in the pan. Cook about four minutes or until it's seared on the outside and not quite done in the middle. Add zoodles and toss to coat with the oil, then spread them out and let cook until they begin to brown.

Add in rest of veggies and turn the heat off. Divide between two plates and top with toasted cashews.

7. Winter Veggie Gratin

Serves 6.

- 3 large spiralized parsnips
- 2 spiralized sweet potatoes
- 1 spiralized butternut squash
- 2 tbsp olive oil
- Salt and pepper
- 2 tbsp butter
- 1 sliced sweet onion
- 1 minced garlic clove
- ¼ cup all-purpose flour
- 1 cup milk
- ¾ cup grated Parmesan
- ¾ cup plus ½ cup grated Gruyere cheese

Preheat oven to 400 degrees and grease a 9x13 casserole dish. Place parsnips, sweet potatoes, and butternut squash in the dish. Drizzle over olive oil and salt and pepper to taste. Toss so veggies are coated and roast 30–35 minutes or until they're tender.

Melt butter over medium heat and cook sweet onion until transparent, about four minutes. Add garlic until fragrant, about one minute. Stir in flour until combined, then add milk and bring to a simmer. Stir in Parmesan and ¾ cup grated Gruyere and season with salt and pepper.

Take the casserole dish out of the oven and pour the sauce over the veggies, tossing to combine. Sprinkle additional ½ cup Gruyere over the top and return to the oven. Bake until cheese is melted and a golden brown color, about 12–15 minutes.

8. Taco Skillet

Serves 6

- 1 tbsp olive oil
- 1 large chopped onion
- 1 lb ground meat (turkey, lean beef, or combo of the two)
- 2 tsp taco seasoning
- Salt
- 4 oz diced green chilies
- 14 oz can diced tomatoes
- 14 oz can rinsed and drained black beans
- 8 corn tortillas
- 1 cup shredded cheddar cheese
- Optional toppings like lettuce, tomatoes, sour cream, avocados, etc. to taste

Swirl olive oil to coat pan in skillet over medium-high heat. Sauté onion for about one minute. Add meat, taco seasoning, and salt. Cook for about seven minutes, stirring and breaking up meat with spatula.

Add green chilies, tomatoes, and black beans; bring to a boil. Cover and simmer on low heat for about five minutes.

On top, place tortillas (they can overlap each other), sprinkle with cheddar cheese. Turn off the heat and make sure it's tightly covered. Let stand for 5–10 minutes.

Add optional toppings if you like.

Shopping list

- Green apple
- Mango
- Blueberries
- Banana
- Frozen pineapple
- Frozen peaches
- Dates
- Raisins
- Spinach
- Baby spinach
- Romaine
- Butter lettuce
- Arugula
- Kale
- Bok choy
- Basil leaves
- Fresh oregano
- Cucumbers
- Persian cucumbers

- Carrots
- Potatoes
- Sweet potatoes
- Red bell pepper
- Yellow bell pepper
- Yellow onion
- Sweet onion
- Red onion
- Broccoli
- Parsnips
- Zucchini
- Butternut squash
- Spaghetti squash
- Cremini mushrooms
- Roasted red peppers
- Kalamata olives
- Ginger
- Jalapeno pepper (optional)
- Cilantro (if applicable)
- Cherry tomatoes
- Beefsteak tomatoes
- Canned fire-roasted tomatoes
- Canned tomato paste
- Can diced chilies
- Garlic
- Limes
- Almond milk or soy milk
- Milk

- Butter
- Olive oil
- Almond butter
- Pine nuts
- Greek yogurt
- Ground turkey
- Lean ground beef
- Skinless, boneless chicken breast
- Skinless, boneless chicken thighs
- Sliced deli ham
- Eggs
- Shrimp
- Flank steak
- Canned kidney beans
- Canned black beans
- Reduced fat shredded cheddar cheese
- Fresh mozzarella
- Parmesan
- Gruyere cheese
- Goat cheese
- Sliced Colby Jack or cheddar cheese
- Cashews
- Mixed nuts
- Oatmeal
- Whole grain tortilla chips
- Whole grain pasta
- Whole grain bread
- Whole grain pita (optional)

- Baguette
- Soba (buckwheat) noodles
- Whole grain rice
- Vanilla extract
- Chili powder
- Cumin
- Cinnamon
- Cocoa powder
- Salt
- Black pepper
- Red pepper flakes
- Smoked paprika
- Taco seasoning
- Fresh thyme
- Dill
- Chives
- Fresh rosemary
- Garlic powder
- Sesame seeds
- Coconut sugar
- Roasted pistachios
- Salsa (or make your own)
- Guacamole
- Light soy sauce/tamari
- Rice wine vinegar
- Balsamic vinegar
- Sesame oil
- Avocado oil

- Honey
- Chicken stock
- Tahini (sesame paste)
- Marinara sauce
- Nutritional yeast

Inspiration: Tom Brady

This athlete is well-known for his prowess on the football field, but also for his clean diet. He drinks a lot of water and aims to reduce inflammation in his body, which means he's cut certain food groups out of his meals entirely, like dairy, sugar and other refined carbs, and caffeine.

Breakfast includes avocado and eggs in addition to a smoothie. Salad with nuts and fish is his go-to lunch dish, and roasted veggies and chicken for dinner. His snacks tend to be full of protein, like hummus and mixed nuts, or with good fats like guacamole. Yet he also allows himself the occasional treat—as long as the food is high quality.

Food for thought

Time to reflect on what you currently have in your kitchen, as well as your eating habits that haven't been working.

- Are you eating enough food: breakfast, lunch, dinner, and snack?
- Are you eating high-quality food at each meal and snack?

- What do you already have in your kitchen that you can use for the 14-day eating plan?
- How will you handle leftovers?
- What do you need to buy in order to make your 14-day plan work?

Chapter Summary

Eating clean doesn't mean a sad salad every day. Not only can salads be tasty and awesome, but you can eat real meals that don't leave you deprived. This two-week plan is just what you need to kickstart your journey to better health in midlife.

8

DON'T FORGET ABOUT YOUR MIND

"You have to think it before you can do it. The mind is what makes it all possible."

— KAI GREENE

You now have a schedule for two weeks for your physical movement as well as what you eat. Missing anything? Yes—the brain you need for healthy weight-loss success.

Have you ever sat down to watch a TV show with a big bag of chips and realized at the end of the show that you've eaten the whole bag? Or maybe you feel nervous or anxious about something, and next thing you know, you're half a carton of ice cream down.

Many people treat food as a reward or even just "something to do," and both of these lead to weight gain. Even when you're eating clean, you won't lose weight when you're hitting the almond butter out of boredom or worry. That's why it's so important to bring your brain into your 14-day reset.

Staying mindful helps you avoid these mind traps and gives you some time to think about whether or not you really need that extra helping of dinner—because you probably don't. When your mind is working on the problem, you'll find the whole body reset much easier to achieve.

What is mindfulness?

You've probably heard about this concept—it's well-known in wellness circles. Basically, what mindfulness boils down to is paying attention to what you're doing while you're doing it. Which sounds pretty simple, and it is. But that doesn't mean it's always easy!

It's the ability to be fully present in the current moment. You're not reacting to or overwhelmed by the world around you, and you're aware of yourself and the space you're in. Also important in mindfulness is the quality of not judging. You may notice things, but you don't attach a judgment to them or try to decide whether they're good or bad or some other value. You simply let everything be as it is.

Human minds like to take flight, which is why mindfulness isn't always easy. But when you notice that your mind is busy thinking about the past or the future, you don't get angry with it for doing something that human brains do, and you don't attach a value judgment to yourself because your mind has sailed away somewhere. You simply gently bring it back to the present moment.

Having said that, it's not always easy; still, anyone can be mindful. Even if you're neurodivergent in some way, or you have several children, or you're trying to juggle work, family, and home. Every human comes equipped with this ability, and it's just a matter of accessing it. Later in the chapter, you'll discover a number of different ways to be mindful because some will probably work better than others.

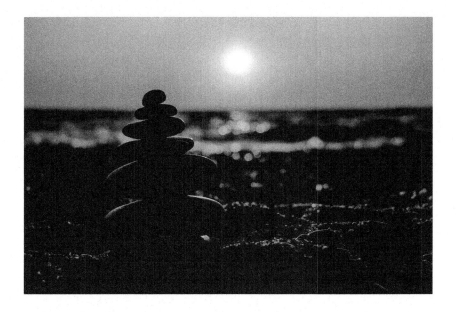

Mindfulness is not something that belongs to certain people. Nor do you have to be a calm or serene type of person for it to work. In fact, the less calm and serene you are, the more you need to practice mindfulness!

It's also not a goal. You can't just wake up one day and say, I have achieved mindfulness! and never practice again. It's more like clean eating and movement: something that you do every day or almost every day that brings you plenty of benefits.

A good mindfulness practice involves both your body and your brain. Many people think that these are two separate parts of the human experience, but in actual fact, both are necessary, and they intertwine. Did you know that you have neurons in your gut, for example? Your brain and body constantly communicate with each other, and tuning into that can help you de-stress and become more mindful.

What's the big deal about mindfulness when it comes to weight loss?

You might recall earlier in the book learning about what our human ancestors needed for survival, and many of those concepts are still "baked into" our brains. Most of us Americans don't have to worry about food scarcity as ancient humans did, but we still have brain pathways that are designed to make sure we eat certain kinds of foods.

Remember how good that chocolate cake tasted when you ate it? Your brain sure does. Not only that, but your brain likes things that make you feel good, so it requests more. More chocolate cake, because sugar is yummy! Or, depending on what your favorite foods are, more French fries (salty) or steak (fatty)!

And the next time you're feeling stressed out, lonely, or bored, or whatever your usual trigger is, your brain remembers the happy time with the cake or fries or steak and wants to replicate that good time. Back you go to the kitchen.

Unfortunately, it's a downward spiral for the habit loops in your brain. The more you reward yourself with food when you face a trigger, the more your brain associates food with soothing that trigger. The neural pathways that link these sensations become stronger over time.

If you've got extra weight, don't blame your tummy—it's your brain that's amplifying the problem. Studies show that mindfulness not only helps people lose weight, but helps them keep it off as well.[1]

Food response and emotions mostly reside in your lizard or reptile brain, which is also responsible for the fight-or-flight (or tend-and-befriend) response to stress. This part of the brain works much faster than the logical part. That's why sometimes you might even feel like you didn't know what came over you, because your reptile brain got to the food before your logical part could say, "Hey, wait, do we really want to do this?"

The logical part of the brain involves what's known as the prefrontal cortex, and it's much bigger in humans than in other animals. This is the part that thinks logically, makes out lists of the pros and cons of a decision, and helps you with spreadsheets or tax returns or other human tasks that animals don't have to deal with.

Your prefrontal cortex is what helps you think about whether or not you really want that chocolate cake, or that second helping of dinner, or the extra-large French fry order. Mindfulness helps build up your prefrontal cortex, so your logical brain is more available to you.

But it also helps you understand why you're reaching for the extra food you don't need. Mindfulness gives you time for a pause to think about whether you want to substitute a healthier alternative than the cake or steak or whether you want to give in to the craving at all, knowing that cravings come and go.

As Charles Duhigg explains in his book, *The Power of Habit*, once habit loops form in your brain, they're almost unbreakable. If you're wondering why you have such a hard time breaking out of your junk food habit, it's not really a question of willpower. It's about the habit loop that you've formed.

While bad habits may not be breakable, they can be changed. The habit loop consists of three parts:

1. Trigger or cue

This is what sets off the habit loop. It can be something tangible like putting your bag on the table, signaling that you're home from work. But it can also be an emotion or an event, like your mom always telling you about how well your older sister is doing and how thin and accomplished she is.

2. Action (habit)

This can be either something healthy or unhealthy. A healthy habit would be to journal about how you feel when you have those calls with your mom or to get on your indoor treadmill when you get home from work.

Or chips and TV time when you get home from work, or downing a pint of ice cream after you get off the phone.

3. Reward

Sometimes this is something tangible, but often it's not. When you're creating a new habit, it's often a good idea to make an explicit reward to help your brain associate your new habit with fun and joy. Like, if you do your half-hour on the treadmill, you get to watch your fave show—but only if you do your treadmill.

After a while, you don't need the explicit rewards because you'll recognize how good you feel after your exercise.

If you're modifying a current habit, you might need to figure out what reward you're getting from the behavior. For example, you might think that eating the ice cream after making a tough phone call doesn't give you a reward—but it absolutely does.

Often, eating comfort food feels good in the moment. And sometimes it helps you become numb to the emotions you're experiencing. You're feeling bad after that phone call, and eating the ice cream helps you forget (at least momentarily) how bad you feel. That's definitely a reward.

The loop itself stays once it's wired into your neural pathways. What you can do is change the action and the reward steps of the loop into something that's healthy.

Suppose one of your bad habits is coming home from work, tossing your coat on the chair, grabbing a bag of chips or a can of beer and heading to your recliner to watch your favorite streaming show. The cue is tossing your coat on the chair, and the current habit is the chips or beer and zoning out in front of the TV. The reward might be a feeling of relaxation, or numbing out, or doing something for yourself instead of everyone else.

If you've decided that habit is keeping you fat (which it is) and you want to change it, figure out what action you'll substitute for your current one. Maybe you want to relax after work, which is completely understandable. What other ways can you relax? Some people like bubble baths, others like to take a walk, and some might want to call a friend.

Or maybe you want to do something just for yourself. You could read if that's enjoyable, do a hobby, or even get on the treadmill with your earbuds in and listen to whatever you want. By switching to a healthy behavior, you might allow yourself non-food treats like bingeing your fave show, or intangible rewards like feeling better in your body and about yourself.

Seems logical, right? But now you're wondering what mindfulness has to do with this. While you're building this new habit of healthy actions, mindfulness can keep you focused on what you're doing so you don't automatically repeat the bad behavior in response to the cue.

You have a little pause that allows you to bring your prefrontal cortex into the mix: Will I be happy in the long run if I eat the chips, or will I feel better taking the dog for a walk? Dog it is. So what should I do now? Put a leash on the pooch and get my walking shoes on.

In particular, mindfulness around food helps you concentrate on what your food looks like, its texture, its scent, and its taste. Ever notice how when you have a cold or allergies, food doesn't taste the same? That's because you can't smell it as well, and the smell heavily influences the taste of your food.

You'll also be better equipped to notice what foods you crave in response to emotions and events, which can help you make better decisions. It allows you to sit with the cravings because there's no judgment when it comes to mindfulness, just noticing what's going on. Cravings will subside when you don't give into them.

Boost mindfulness while you're eating by adapting your environment

Do you know why most fast-food places feature the colors red and yellow? Because they make people eat faster. It takes some time for the "I'm full" signals of the belly to reach your brain—about 20 minutes. If you eat faster than that, you may still feel hungry and need to go back for more.

Being mindful as you eat helps you slow down and actually taste your food. There are a number of ways to help you focus on eating so you can stay present and allow the full belly signals to reach your brain before you end up eating too much.

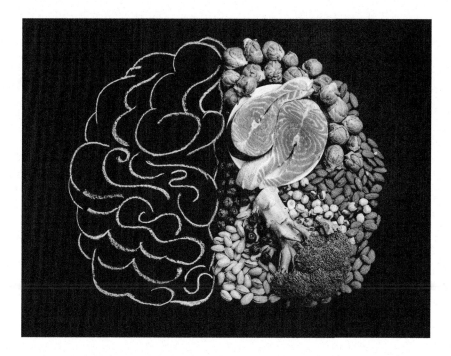

- Turn off your electronics

Don't distract yourself from your food—it's too easy to eat way too much when you're not paying attention. Leave the TV off, and if you can't bring yourself to leave your phone in a different room, which is best, at least turn it face down on the table.

If you have kids, family meals are a great time to bond and find out what your kids are up to. It's also good for them to take regular breaks away from their phones. They might not be happy about it at first, and that's okay. You're the parent, not their friend or sibling.

Even if you don't have kids, being able to focus on your food will help you stop eating when you're done. (You could also use a break from your phone.)

- Sit down at a table

When you're catching food on the run, you're not going to be able to concentrate. Eating in the car means you have no idea how full you are because your attention is elsewhere. You can't enjoy your food when you're wolfing it down as you zoom down the freeway. Yes, it's more convenient to eat on the move, but do you want to lose weight or not?

- Chew your food slowly

You get the chance to enjoy your food when you can really taste it, as opposed to gulping it down. And you may find that the entire piece of chocolate cake, or the entire steak, doesn't taste as good. The first few bites are bliss, but after that, not so much. Really get the flavor from your food by chewing slowly.

Once you've stopped eating so many fast-food meals and you've started creating flavorful meals from scratch, you'll find that you can really taste good food again. Your mouth hasn't been blasted away by the sugar/fat/salt bomb, and now you can savor the flavors.

- Determine the good places in your area to eat out

Although most of your food should come from your kitchen, there are going to be some days and nights when that is just not realistic. Or you want to celebrate something with a meal that you didn't make yourself (and don't have to clean up!)

Map out restaurants that feature whole foods or that don't have as many fried items on the menu. Ones that have an assortment of tasty salads and vegetable-based dishes are good. Many cuisines from outside the US, like Thai or Indian, don't have a lot of fried or heavy meat-based dishes, so those restaurants can be good choices.

Maybe there's a place that serves your favorite entree exactly the way you like it or one that makes a dessert that you love. It'll taste even better when you haven't had it for a while, and your taste buds aren't used to it.

You should probably skip the usual fast-food and "fast casual" chain restaurants most of the time. They tend to feature a lot of fried food in huge servings, which is not what you need for a celebration or a nice meal out.

Helpful mindful habits for everyday life

Meditation doesn't necessarily mean having to sit down for an hour and force yourself to think about nothing—even though that's a popular myth. Meditation itself has numerous benefits, and there are different ways to practice it.

However, in all practices, it's common for the mind to wander off. Remember, it's all about no judgment, so just bring your mind gently back to the meditation. If you find that sitting down and being still is too difficult, or you're in a place where it won't work, you can also try mindful walking and mindful breathing.

Meditation itself is just a way for you to learn how to focus your mind and redirect your thoughts. Prayer can be a form of meditation, so you might already be practicing it. And meditation is a practice—like mindfulness, it's not a goal to achieve but something that you do on a regular basis. When you practice consistently, that's when you'll notice the results.

There are two main avenues for meditation. One is a focused practice, where you focus on a single thought, object, sound, or visualization. This includes mantras and breathing meditations and is designed to help you get rid of distractions.

Note that thoughts will pop up—that's what the human brain does. That doesn't mean you're bad at meditation, or you can't do it, because this happens to everyone. You'll learn how to stay detached from thoughts (and feelings that may arise) and let them go.

The other type of practice is open-monitoring, where you are aware of everything that's going on around you as well as your thoughts and your being. This is a good way to uncover thoughts or feelings that you've been suppressing.

Meditation has a variety of benefits. If you're not already convinced, this is something to add to your life!

1. Improves anxiety

Meditation is an effective way to control anxiety, particularly if you have high levels of it. It helps people cope with their lives and improves resiliency to things that might otherwise stress them out.

2. Reduces stress

Trying to reduce stress is one of the main reasons that people try meditation. Mindfulness meditation (which we'll get into in the next section) specifically has been shown to decrease the inflammation that comes along with stress.[2]

3. Decreases blood pressure

High blood pressure makes your heart work harder than it needs to and narrows your arteries, which leads to cardiovascular disease, including strokes. Meditation can help relax the nerve signals around heart function, the tension in your blood vessels, and the stress response.[3]

4. Improves emotional health

Because meditation, especially mindfulness meditation, can help you improve your self-image, you'll get an emotional health boost from your practice.

5. Boosts self-awareness

When you understand yourself better, you can then create the best version of yourself. Certain forms of meditation help you recognize negative or defeatist thoughts, so you can then develop a more constructive version of those thoughts.

6. May increase kindness

Not just to others, but to yourself as well. Loving-kindness meditation helps you get better at being kind to yourself. Once you can be kind to yourself, you can then extend it to others.

This can be especially helpful in midlife, when you've got some extra weight and may feel bad about yourself. So many of us have a tendency to beat ourselves up! But has that worked? If you've been unkind to yourself about your weight and you're still overweight, that tells you that being unkind isn't going to help you drop the weight.

7. May help with memory loss

When you're able to pay attention and think clearly, you may help prevent age-related memory loss or dementia. It's all about keeping your brain young. Just as exercise helps your body stay flexible and strong, so too can meditation help your brain stay flexible and stronger for longer.

8. Increases attention span

At mid-life, so many Americans (especially women) feel pulled in multiple directions. You may find that you start things and are unable to finish them due to a shortened attention span. If that's something that bothers you, focused meditation can help! You'll learn to increase your attention span and make it stronger at the same time.

9. May help with addictions

With the discipline that comes from meditation, you'll be more aware of your triggers and be better able to control yourself around them. You'll learn to redirect your focus and possibly understand the causes of the addiction. Then you can address them and find healthy coping mechanisms.

10. Improves pain

So much of pain is in your brain, and when you're stressed out, things can feel more painful than otherwise. It not only helps decrease people cope better with their pain but can also help reduce the symptoms of chronic pain.

11. Improves sleep

Insomnia, or problems sleeping, often get better with meditation practice. You learn to deal with racing thoughts, plus you'll feel more relaxed.

Now that you understand some of the intense positive effects of meditation, let's talk techniques. Just as you can't expect flawless performance the first time you dance, you probably won't be able to meditate for 15–20 minutes right away.

Meditation practice is also similar to exercise in that a little is better than none. Start with just five minutes at first. After that begins to feel easy, you can start adding a little more time, maybe 10 minutes, and so on.

Find a time of day that you won't be interrupted, or at least less likely to be interrupted, because this is about you and not anyone else. You can meditate anywhere at any time, so choose a time and place where you can be consistent about your practice at first.

At this stage of life, you're probably used to caring for other people or putting them first. That's not necessarily a bad thing! But when you go on the airplane and the flight attendant starts talking about the oxygen masks, what do they say? They tell you to put your own oxygen mask first.

Why is that? Well, if you can't breathe, you can't help anyone else. Putting your own mask on first is the only way that you can help others. Meditation is a time for you to work on you so that you can then help others. You can't pour from an empty cup, so fill your cup first.

- Meditation

There are a lot of techniques for meditation, so the ones listed here for beginners aren't the only ones you can try. You might immediately decide from the descriptions that you want to try a certain type. But if not, don't worry about it–pick one and give it a go. Give your practice at least a week or two while you're meditating every day to see how you feel about it. You will get more benefits from meditating for longer than five minutes, so if you're not seeing all the benefits, you might just want to increase your time spent each day.

- Mindfulness

In this type of meditation, you'll be focusing on what you're feeling or sensing in each moment– no judgment and no interpretation. You might focus on your breath and how it feels (more about mindful breathing later), or do a body scan where you slowly survey your body from the crown of your head to the tips of your toes.

- Focus

Here you pay close attention to some object, which could be a flower, a candle, or some memento. You examine each aspect of it so closely that there's no room for anything else. Objects that have other senses tied to them, like a rose or scented candle that you can smell, work well.

If you chose a candle, for example, you would sit comfortably in front of it and study the flame and how it flickers and what colors it's made of, how the wax drips down the sides or pools in the bottom, the sounds of the candle burning and its scent, and so forth.

Great for building a better attention span.

- Mantra

You repeat a word or a phrase a certain number of times, like 108 times as is traditional. It could be a word like peace or love, or it could be "ohm," or anything else. You can repeat it out loud or say it in your head. If you like, you can count on beads or a mala.

The repetition helps you focus and ignore distractions. You can add breathing to the mantra so that you breathe in on the first syllable and out on the second.

- Progressive relaxation

Here you focus on tightening and then releasing muscles, typically either working your way up from your feet or down from your head. This is a good one to do in bed and can help calm you and get you ready for sleep.

As you tighten and relax your muscles, you focus on the ones that you're working on, rather than thinking about your day or anything else.

- Guided

These types of meditations are often great for beginners, as they often involve visualizations or imagery so your mind has something to do. Many of them are available on apps or YouTube.

One visualization that you can try if you don't want to listen to a guided meditation is the beach walk. Close your eyes. In your mind, put yourself on a beautiful beach. Listen to the sounds, smell the surf, taste the briny water in addition to looking at the fine sand and the waves.

If you'd like to listen to some soothing music, there are plenty of resources available. You might try tracks from some of the following:

- Music for Body and Spirit
- Well+ Good's Music for Meditation
- Classic FM's Classical Meditation Music

- Mindful walking

This is meditation while you're moving. You're aware of how your body and mind feel as you walk as well as the environment around you. You should do this practice for at least 10 minutes, and it should also be done outside in a natural setting, so you get the benefits of being outdoors too.

Stand still a few minutes before you start walking, breathing, and grounding yourself. Feel your entire body. As you start walking, pay attention to your movements and how they feel in your body. Notice how you carry yourself and the position of your head, chest, arms, legs, and feet. How do they feel as you go?

Once you're comfortable with the sensations of your body, you can open up your focus to include the area around you. When thoughts come in, as they will, kindly and gently, without any judgment, bring your mind back to your body and its movements. You might choose to focus on your feet or your breath, or some other area with a lot of sensation.

After your walk, take time to notice how you feel. Refreshed? Calm? Energized? Something else?

• Mindful breathing

Your breath is always with you, so it's a good thing to anchor on when you're meditating. If during the day you feel yourself stressing or spiraling, your breath is there to help you de-stress. Plus, no one else necessarily needs to know what you're doing. It can be done standing up, though sitting or lying down is even better.

If you need some mindful breaths during a suddenly stressful time during the day, try a simple technique like deeply inhaling through your nose for three counts, holding at the top for two counts, then exhaling through your mouth for four counts.

You could also try box breathing: in for four counts, hold for four counts, exhale for four counts, and hold for four counts. Slowing down your breathing assures your body that you are not threatened and don't need to be in flight-or-flight mode, so the brain and body will turn off stress responses.

When practicing for longer periods, find yourself a comfortable position, sitting with your back straight but not rigid. You might close your eyes or let your gaze rest softly on the floor. Notice the chair or seat you're on and the sensations of your body on it.

Then, notice your breath. You don't need to change it in any way, just notice the sensations as you breathe in and out in your nose, chest, stomach, and wherever else the breath moves you. Keep noticing. When thoughts intrude, as they do, gently return your focus to your breath once you notice your mind got carried away. No judgment, no attachment. Just back to the breath.

Do this for 5–7 minutes (set a timer). At the end, notice again the seat where you're sitting and any other body sensations, then give yourself a little thanks for taking the time to do this.

Inspiration: Tracee Ellis Ross

Known for her TV roles, especially on the show Black-ish, Tracee Ellis Ross relaxes through meditation. During the COVID-19 pandemic, she converted her meditation room to a home gym—but not for the reason you might think.

She recognized that she didn't need to carve out just one space for it. She sets out items that bring her joy, like a jade pig she bought on a trip to Thailand with her mother. Her whole home is a place to meditate.

Food for thought

You might think differently about meditation now that you understand the many benefits and techniques you can use.

- When and where is a good time and space for you to set up a meditation practice?
- What technique spoke to you, and if none did, which will you try first?
- How can you make the space welcoming and comfortable so that you look forward to your meditation time?

Chapter Summary

Now you've got all the tools you need for a whole body reset. This book will be here for you whenever you need to refresh your memory, or maybe try a different recipe or mindfulness technique when you need more motivation.

---

1. https://www.aarp.org/health/healthy-living/info-2019/mindfulness-weight-loss.html
2. http://www.healthline.com/nutrition/12-benefits-of-meditation
3. Ibid.

9

MORE RECIPES

"Ability is what you're capable of doing. Motivation determines what you do. Attitude determines how well you do it."

— LOU HOLTZ

The Whole Body Reset is a way for you to start your journey toward better health in midlife. But once you're past the fourteen days, you might want some more variety in your meals. Or there may have been a recipe earlier in the book that doesn't work for your dietary restrictions. Here are some more recipes that you can swap in for any of the ones on your 14-day plan.

Detox smoothies (serves 1 unless otherwise noted)

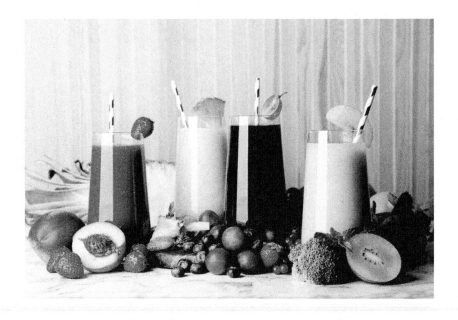

1. Blueberry

- 1 cup frozen wild blueberries
- 1 small handful fresh cilantro
- 1 cut-up frozen banana
- ¼ avocado
- ½ cup orange juice
- ½ cup water

Blend together and serve.

2. Pineapple grapefruit

Serves 2.

- 1 peeled and sectioned red grapefruit
- 2 cups frozen pineapple
- ⅓ cup Greek yogurt
- 1 tbsp coconut oil
- ¼ inch section peeled fresh ginger
- Optional toppings: granola, grapefruit segments, and berries

Blend first five ingredients. If you like, top with granola, grapefruit segments, and berries to serve.

3. Banana kale

- 2 cups unsweetened coconut milk
- 2 tsp matcha green tea powder
- 2 frozen cut-up bananas
- 1 handful baby kale
- 1 tsp honey

Blend together and serve.

4. Liver helper

- 1 ripe peeled banana
- ½ cored apple
- 1 peeled medium-size carrot (cut up)
- 1 handful baby spinach
- ¼ inch section peeled fresh turmeric
- 1 tbsp chopped parsley
- 3 walnut halves
- 2 tbsp protein powder
- juice of ½ lemon
- pinch cinnamon
- ¾ cup almond milk

Blend together until smooth and serve.

5. Green Glow

- 1 banana
- 1 kiwi
- ¼ cup pineapple
- 2 celery stalks
- 2 cups spinach
- 1 cup water

Blend all ingredients until smooth.

Lunches

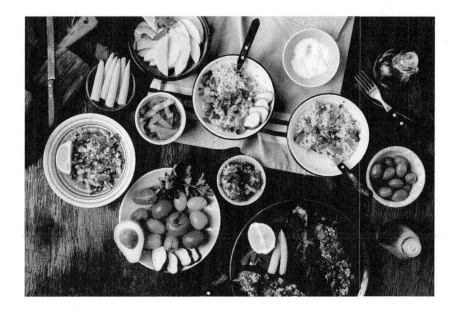

1. Easy Chicken Gyros

Serves 6.

For chicken marinade:

- 2 lbs chicken breast cut into cubes
- ¼ cup plus ½ tbsp olive oil
- 3 plus 2 crushed garlic cloves
- Juice of 1 lemon
- 3 tbsp chopped parsley
- 1½ tbsp dried oregano
- ½ tbsp dried mint
- 1 tsp salt

- ½ teaspoon black pepper
- 3 bay leaves

For tzatziki:

- ½ peeled cucumber
- 1 cup Greek yogurt
- 2 crushed garlic cloves
- 2 tsp lemon juice (about ¼ lemon)
- 1½ tbsp chopped fresh dill
- ½ tbsp olive oil
- ¼ teaspoon salt
- pinch black pepper

For serving (vegetables and cheese to taste):

- 6 pitas
- Romaine lettuce
- Chopped tomatoes
- Chopped red onion
- Chopped cucumber
- Feta cheese

Combine chicken marinade ingredients. Refrigerate at least 10 minutes to overnight.

Meanwhile, make tzatziki: grate cucumber through cheese-cloth and set drained cuke in a bowl. Mix with Greek yogurt,

2 crushed garlic cloves, ½ tbsp olive oil, lemon juice, dill, salt and pepper. Refrigerate at least 1 hour.

Grill chicken to taste, with internal temperature at least 165 degrees.

Warm 6 pitas on the grill, then add romaine lettuce, chopped tomatoes, red onion, cucumber, and crumbled feta cheese down the middle of each pita. Top with chicken and generous scoop of tzatziki and fold in half to serve.

2. Vegan hummus wrap

Serves 1.

- 1 wheat tortilla (if you like) or lettuce leaf
- ½ cup hummus
- 1 sliced mini cucumber
- ½ sliced tomato
- ½ sliced small avocado
- 1 cup mixed greens
- Alfalfa and microgreens if desired

Heat tortilla and spread with hummus. Layer on cucumber, tomato, and avocado. Top with greens. Roll up to serve.

3. Korean Steak Rice Bowl

Serves 2.

For steak marinade:

- 1 lb. sirloin or flank steak cut into 2-inch strips
- 2 tbsp soy sauce
- 2 tbsp brown sugar
- 2 tsp vegetable oil
- 2 tsp sesame oil, divided in half
- 1 tsp each ground black pepper, ginger, minced garlic, and cornstarch

For veggies:

- ½ cup broccoli florets
- ⅓ cup shredded carrots
- ¼ cup chopped chives
- ⅓ cup bean sprouts
- 1 tbsp each soy sauce, rice vinegar, water, and sugar
- 1 chopped, peeled potato
- ⅔ cup steamed rice
- Kimchi
- Garnish: green onion, sesame seeds

Combine steak marinade ingredients. Refrigerate at least 30 minutes or overnight.

Meanwhile, bring one pot of water to a boil. Turn off heat and add broccoli, carrots, chives, and bean sprouts. Blanch one minute and drain. Mix soy sauce, rice vinegar, water, and sugar with 1 tsp. sesame oil. Add veggies and let sit 10–15 minutes.

Bring one pot water to boil and add potato and cook 6–7 minutes only. Drain.

Heat skillet over medium-high heat and stir-fry beef and potatoes for about seven minutes or until beef browns. Lower heat and cover; cook additional minute.

To each bowl, add ⅓ cup steamed rice. Top with ½ beef and potatoes mixture, ½ veggie mixture, and kimchi to taste. Garnish if you like with green onions and sesame seeds.

4. Coconut curry lentil soup

Serves 4–6.

- 1¼ cups dry brown lentils
- 1 tbsp coconut oil
- ½ cup chopped onion
- 2 minced garlic cloves
- 1 tbsp grated ginger
- ¼ tsp turmeric
- 2 tsp garam masala
- ½ tbsp yellow curry powder
- 1 tsp cumin

- 2 medium carrots peeled and chopped
- 1 tbsp tomato paste
- 2 cups vegetable broth
- 1 can coconut milk
- Salt and pepper

Prepare lentils by pouring over boiling water. Let sit 10 minutes.

Heat coconut oil over medium heat and add onion, garlic, ginger, and turmeric. Sauté 2–3 minutes or until onions are translucent, then add garam masala, curry powder, and cumin and cook another minute.

Stir in prepared lentils, carrots, potato, tomato paste, 1½ cups water, vegetable broth, and coconut milk. Bring to boil, then reduce to low heat, cover and simmer 15 minutes.

Remove one cup to blend, then add back to pot. Season with salt and pepper to taste.

5. Vegan soba salad

Serves 2–3.

For dressing:

- 1 tbsp each tahini, soy sauce, black rice vinegar
- 1 tsp minced garlic
- ½ tsp ground black pepper

For salad:

- 6 oz. buckwheat soba noodles, about 1½ cups
- 1 cup each thinly shredded red cabbage, peeled and shredded carrots, and cucumber
- ¼ finely chopped cilantro
- 1 tsp. sesame seeds

Bring pot of water to boil over medium-high heat, add noodles and cook 7–8 minutes. Stir occasionally to keep noodles separate, then rinse with cold water and drain.

Whisk all dressing ingredients together in small bowl for about one minute.

Add noodles and salad ingredients to large bowl and toss with dressing to coat.

Snacks

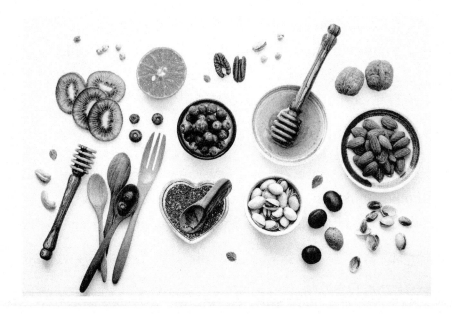

1. Avocado toast with nutritional yeast

Toast your favorite whole wheat bread and spread with smashed avocado. Top with 1 tbsp nutritional yeast.

2. Chocolate chia pudding

Serves 2.

- 2 tbsp chia seeds
- 1 cup almond milk
- 1 tbsp each flaxseed, cacao powder, and brown rice syrup

Mix chia seeds with almond milk with a fork so seeds are evenly distributed. Stir in flaxseed, cacao, and brown rice syrup. Refrigerate at least 30 minutes to overnight.

3. Almond cookies

Serves 6.

- 1 cup almonds
- ½ cup almond butter
- 1 cup pitted dates
- 1¼ tsp vanilla extract

In food processor, blend all ingredients until you have a dough of sorts. Roll into balls and refrigerate 30 minutes.

4. Overnight oats

- ½ cup oats
- 1 cup almond milk
- 3 tbsp protein powder
- 3 almonds
- Optional: ½ mashed banana

Mix first four ingredients in a container and let sit overnight in the refrigerator. If you want it sweeter, add the banana.

5. Spiced nuts

Serves 6.

- 1 cup each raw unsalted almonds, cashews, and walnuts
- ½ cup raw unsalted sunflower seeds
- 2 tsp. smoked paprika
- 1 tsp. salt
- ½ tsp. garlic powder
- 1 tbsp. olive or avocado oil

Preheat oven to 350. Line a baking sheet with parchment paper and place nuts on the sheet in a single layer. Roast 15 minutes, turning halfway through.

Meanwhile, mix spices in a small bowl.

Remove nuts from oven and allow to cool. Toss with oil, then coat with spice mixture. Store in an airtight container at room temperature.

Dinners

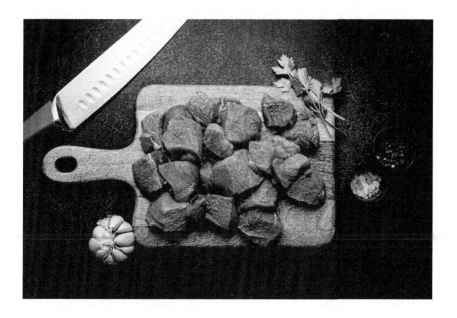

1. Hearty Chickpea and Spinach Stew

Serves 4.

- 2 cans drained and rinsed chickpeas
- 12 oz ground turkey
- ½ tsp. each dried oregano, crushed fennel seeds, and crushed red pepper
- 1 chopped onion
- 2 peeled and diced carrots
- 4 cloves minced garlic
- 3 tbsp tomato paste
- 4 cups chicken broth (1 32-oz carton)

- ¼ tsp ground pepper
- ⅛ tsp salt
- 3 cups frozen spinach, thawed and drained
- 4 tbsp Parmesan cheese

Mash one can of chickpeas and set aside.

Heat oil over medium-high heat and add turkey and oregano, fennel seeds, and red pepper. Cook, separating meat, until no longer pink. Add onion, carrots, and garlic. Cook, stirring often, 3–4 minutes, then add tomato paste and stir for 30 seconds.

Add broth, both cans of chickpeas, ground pepper and salt. Cover and bring to simmer, then lower heat to brisk simmer, covered, for 10 minutes.

Add frozen spinach, increase heat back to medium-high and cook 1–2 minutes or until spinach is hot. Ladle and top each bowl with 1 tbsp. Parmesan cheese, if desired.

2. Roasted Salmon Caprese

Serves 4.

- 1½ tsp olive oil
- 1 grated clove garlic
- ¼ tsp each salt and pepper, twice
- 2 cups quartered cherry tomatoes
- 1 lb. salmon, cut into 4 pieces

- 1 cup halved pearl mozzarella balls
- ¼ cup thinly sliced basil
- 2 tsp. balsamic glaze

Preheat oven to 425 degrees. Coat baking sheet with cooking spray. Stir olive oil, garlic, and salt and pepper together. Toss with cherry tomatoes.

Arrange salmon on one side of baking sheet. Sprinkle with salt and pepper. Cover with mozzarella. Place tomato mixture on other side and bake until salmon just cooked and tomatoes melting, 8–10 minutes.

Stir basil into tomato mixture, then divide over salmon pieces. Drizzle with balsamic glaze.

3. Spinach and Feta-Stuffed Mushrooms

Serves 4.

- 3 tbsp olive oil
- 1 bunch sliced green onions
- 2 minced garlic cloves
- 1 10-oz frozen spinach package, thawed and drained
- ½ cup plus 1 tbsp feta cheese
- ¼ cup chopped dill
- ¼ tsp ground black pepper
- ⅛ tsp salt
- 4 portobello mushrooms (stems and gills removed)

- Crushed pepper, if desired

Preheat oven to 400 degrees. Heat 2 tbsp olive oil in skillet over medium heat, then add green onions and garlic. Cook until soft, about 2–3 minutes, then remove from heat. Stir in spinach, ½ cup feta cheese, dill, ground black pepper, and salt.

Brush portobello mushrooms (stems and gills removed) with 1 tbsp olive oil, place on baking sheet, and stuff with spinach mixture. Bake until hot and beginning to brown, about 15–20 minutes. Sprinkle with 1 tbsp feta, and crushed pepper if desired.

4. Summer Veggie and Egg Scramble

Serves 4.

- 2 tbsp olive oil
- 12 oz. thinly sliced baby potatoes
- 4 cups thinly sliced veggies of your choice (use scraps!)
- 3 green onions, separated into green and white parts
- 1 tsp minced herbs such as rosemary and thyme
- 6 large beaten eggs
- 2 packed cups leafy greens
- ½ tsp salt

Heat olive oil over medium heat and add potatoes. Cook until they soften, about eight minutes. Add veggies and chopped whites of green onions. Cook 8–10 minutes or until veggies are lightly browned, then stir in herbs. Scoot to edges of skillet and add eggs and green parts of green onions to middle of the pan.

Cook, stirring, until eggs are lightly scrambled, about two minutes. Stir greens into eggs, then remove from heat and stir to combine. Stir in salt.

5. Spicy Chicken Soup

Serves 8.

- 1 4-lb. chicken, innards removed
- 1 large yellow onion, peeled and roughly chopped
- 2 roughly chopped carrots
- 2 roughly chopped celery stalks
- 1 large head garlic, cut crosswise
- ½-1 jalapeno pepper (plus more for garnish) cut lengthwise
- 2 3-inch peeled and chopped pieces of ginger
- 1 bunch parsley (plus more for garnish)
- 1 tbsp each coriander seeds and salt
- 2 tsp ground black pepper
- 6 oz mixed greens
- 2 thinly sliced lemons

Combine first ten ingredients in a large pot and cover with water. Cover the pot, bring to a boil, then reduce to a simmer. Cook about one hour, skimming off impurities periodically.

Transfer chicken to a plate and strain the leftover stock into another pot. Keep warm; taste and add salt if necessary. Shred the chicken and freeze additional servings if you like.

Divide greens, jalapeno, chicken, and lemons between serving bowls and top with broth.

LOG YOUR RESET

"Believe in yourself. You are braver than you think, more talented than you know, and capable of more than you imagine."

Roy T. Bennett

I t's a great idea, especially at first, to keep track of your weight and your new habits: how long you meditated/danced/stretched for, which recipes you tried and whether or not you liked them. You can use this tracker or create your own.

Day	Ate clean?	Stretching time	Dancing time	Meditation time	Recipes I liked
1					
2					
3					
4					
5					
6					
7					
8					
9					
10					
11					
12					
13					
14					

Weight day 1:	
Weight day 7:	
Weight day 14:	

CONCLUSION

The good news is that you now have everything you need to jumpstart your journey to healthy living in midlife. You have the tools and resources, and now you just need to put the pieces into place. You've read plenty of success stories throughout the book, and it's time for you to start your own success story!

You learned about aging and its effects on the body and mind, especially in midlife. Fortunately, clean eating and exercise will help prevent or delay many of these symptoms. A long, healthy life is possible when you make the right decisions.

You discovered not only the health benefits of stretching and dance routines but also some techniques and ways to get started. When it comes to movement, it's important to start where you are right now, not where you were 20 years ago or where you want to be. Be gentle and nonjudgemental as you start implementing your flexibility and dancing.

Another major aspect of a healthy midlife journey is clean eating, with lots of unprocessed, whole foods. You now have some recipes and an eating plan to get started, as well as the rules of clean eating. And of course, the occasional celebration with cake or alcohol is part of the plan—after your healthy detox.

The last key component is to ensure that you have the right mindset for success. Being mindful helps prevent you from eating too much food—clean or otherwise—and meditation techniques can also help you stress less. Once you no longer need to eat for comfort or to relieve anxiety, you'll find sticking to your clean eating plan isn't as difficult as you might have thought.

This book will always be here if you need to refresh yourself on any of the principles or even if you need a little motivation to keep going. Don't be afraid to revisit these ideas, especially after your 14-day reset, to ensure that you keep your new good habits in place.

So what are you waiting for? Cue up your dance music playlist and hit the grocery store to buy your healthy, clean foods!

LEAVE A 1-CLICK REVIEW!

I would be incredibly thankful if you could take just 60 seconds to write a brief review on Amazon, even if it's just a few sentences!

If you enjoyed the book and found it helpful, please leave a review. We want to spread the midlife health message to as many people as we can. Thank you!

To leave a quick review just scan the QR code below!

JUST FOR YOU

A FREE GIFT TO OUR READERS

07 amazing recipes to be warm and healthy and enjoy the cold days among family and friends!

WARM & HEALTHY WINTER WITH DELICIOUS SOUPS!

Download here:

PAGEWESTPUBLISHING.COM/GIFT

REFERENCES

Ademarsh, A. (2022a, March 2). Bridge Pose. Retrieved from https://www.yogajournal.com/poses/bridge-pose/

Ademarsh, A. (2022b, March 2). Extended Triangle Pose. Retrieved from https://www.yogajournal.com/poses/extended-triangle-pose/

Ademarsh, A. (2022c, July 26). Warrior 2 Pose. Retrieved from https://www.yogajournal.com/poses/warrior-ii-pose/

Aldecoa, K. (2022, February 18). This Is Jennifer Lopez's Exact Breakfast, Lunch, and Dinner. Retrieved from https://www.eatthis.com/news-jennifer-lopez-diet/

Ball, M. J. S. (2022, June 23). 29 Days of Clean Eating Recipes. Retrieved from https://www.eatingwell.com/gallery/7832853/30-days-of-clean-eating-recipes/

Bel Marra Health. (2017, May 2). Detoxing is Good for Better Digestion. Retrieved from https://www.belmarrahealth.com/detoxing-how-good-is-it-for-better-digestion/

Bjarnadottir, A. (2017, June 4). Why Refined Carbs Are Bad For You. Retrieved from https://www.healthline.com/nutrition/why-refined-carbs-are-bad

Bodybuilding.com. (n.d.). Cross-body shoulder stretch | Exercise Videos & Guides. Retrieved from https://www.bodybuilding.com/exercises/shoulder-stretch

Booth, J. (2020, April 16). 5 Triceps Stretches to Loosen Up Those Arms. Retrieved from https://greatist.com/health/triceps-stretches

Bustos, L. (2021, June 1). How to Do a Frog Stretch Correctly—and Safely. Retrieved from https://www.thehealthy.com/exercise/frog-stretch/

CDC. (2022a, June 2). Move More; Sit Less. Retrieved from https://www.cdc.gov/physicalactivity/basics/adults/index.htm

CDC. (2022b, July 15). Heart Disease Facts | cdc.gov. Retrieved from https://www.cdc.gov/heartdisease/facts.htm

Celestine, N. (2022, July 2). What Is Mindful Breathing? Exercises, Scripts, and Videos. Retrieved from https://positivepsychology.com/mindful-breathing/

Ceres Organic. (2016, July 20). 20 clean eating snacks for people on the run. Retrieved from https://ceres.co.nz/blog/20-clean-eating-snacks-for-busy-people-on-the-run/

Chakraborty, D. (2022, November 17). 10 Fabulously Fit Celebrities over 40 Who Will Inspire You to Embrace Healthy Living Today. Retrieved from https://www.vagabomb.com/Fit-Celebrities-over-40/

Champion, L. (2017, March 8). 30 Easy Clean-Eating Lunches to Try This Month. Retrieved from https://www.purewow.com/food/clean-eating-lunch-recipes

Change to Chill. (2020, July 31). What Is Mindful Walking? Retrieved from https://www.changetochill.org/stay-grounded-with-mindful-walking/

ClassPass. (n.d.). How to do Seated Spinal Twist. Retrieved from https://class pass.com/movements/seated-spinal-twist

Cooking Light. (2020, February 7). 25 Clean Eating Recipes for Weeknights. Retrieved from https://www.cookinglight.com/eating-smart/smart-choices/clean-eating-recipes

Cronkleton, E. (2020, January 17). How to Do a Better Butterfly Stretch. Retrieved from https://www.healthline.com/health/butterfly-stretch

Cronkleton, E. (2021, November 4). 5 Benefits of Frog Pose. Retrieved from https://www.healthline.com/health/fitness/frog-pose-benefits

Davis, N. (2021, June 2). The 90/90 Stretch Can Improve Pain and Function in Your Hips and Back. Retrieved from https://www.healthline.com/health/fitness/90-90-stretch

Drillinger, M. (2020, April 3). Most Diets Don't Work for Weight Loss After a Year: Here's Why. Retrieved from https://www.healthline.com/health-news/diets-work-for-one-year#How-to-fight-back

Duhigg, C. (2014). *The Power of Habit: Why We Do What We Do in Life and Business*. New York, NY: Random House Trade Paperbacks.

Dumain, T. (2018, January 4). How to Stretch Your Neck. Retrieved from https://www.webmd.com/fitness-exercise/fitness-neck-stretches

Dutter, E. (2019, September 18). Clean eating: What does that mean? Retrieved from https://www.mayoclinichealthsystem.org/hometown-health/speaking-of-health/clean-eating-what-does-that-mean

Fargo, M., & Heath, C. (2022, July 27). 41 celebrity food, fitness and sleep habits to steal. Retrieved from https://www.womenshealthmag.com/uk/food/healthy-eating/g27164610/celebrity-health-habits/

Fink, R. (n.d.). Gaining Weight in Your 40s: Facts and Tips – Miami Center of Excellence | Dr. Randy Fink – Miami OBGYNS. Retrieved from https://www.miamiobgyns.com/blog/gaining-weight-in-your-40s-facts-and-tips-mcoe/

Fitnut Loft. (n.d.). 6 Reasons Why Women Gain Weight After 40. Retrieved from https://fitnutloft.com/blog/129172/6-Reasons-Why-Women-Gain-Weight-After-40

Four Sail Collaboration. (2020, July 20). Get Moore in Shape: Demi Moore's Diet and Fitness Tips. Retrieved from https://www.onebodyonelife.com/blogs/blog/get-moore-in-shape-demi-moores-diet-and-fitness-tips

Fuentes, L. (2021, April 14). 10 Best Clean Eating Snacks. Retrieved from https://www.laurafuentes.com/clean-eating-snacks/

Gilmore, M. (2022, July 1). Easy Detox Smoothie (with NO weird ingredients!). Retrieved from https://detoxinista.com/detox-smoothie/

Greater Good In Action. (n.d.). Mindful Breathing (Greater Good in Action). Retrieved from https://ggia.berkeley.edu/practice/mindful_breathing

Gunnars, K. (2018, May 4). 10 Leading Causes of Weight Gain and Obesity. Retrieved from https://www.healthline.com/nutrition/10-causes-of-weight-gain#TOC_TITLE_HDR_2

Hartel, K. (n.d.). 11 Reasons You Should Be Eating More Beans / Nutrition / Tips. Retrieved from https://www.fitday.com/fitness-articles/nutrition/tips/11-reasons-you-should-be-eating-more-beans.html

Harvard Health. (2021, April 12). What is inflammation? Retrieved from https://www.health.harvard.edu/heart-disease/ask-the-doctor-what-is-inflammation

Harvard Health. (2022, March 14). The importance of stretching. Retrieved from https://www.health.harvard.edu/staying-healthy/the-importance-of-stretching

Heart.org. (2022, June 2). What is Cholesterol? Retrieved from https://www.heart.org/en/health-topics/cholesterol/about-cholesterol

Helmer, J. (2020, August 2). Dancing for Exercise: Ballroom, Hip Hop, Latin, and More. Retrieved from https://www.webmd.com/fitness-exercise/a-z/dance-for-exercise

Iosune, I. (2019, May 22). Detox Smoothie. Retrieved from https://simpleveg

anblog.com/detox-smoothie/

Jefit. (n.d.). Standing Bicep Stretch. Retrieved from https://www.jefit.com/exercises/806/standing-biceps-stretch

Julian, J. (2020, October 12). Tracee Ellis Ross's Approach to Meditation Is All About What Brings You Joy. Retrieved from https://www.yahoo.com/video/tracee-ellis-rosss-approach-meditation-223928180.html

K. (2021, August 12). 30 Clean Eating Recipes You'll Actually Want to Eat. Retrieved from https://iowagirleats.com/30-clean-eating-recipes/

Kang, W. (2022, June 8). How to Do a Figure 4 Stretch. Retrieved from https://www.beachbodyondemand.com/blog/figure-4-stretch

Kennedy, S. (2022, March 29). How Mindfulness Can Impact Weight Loss. Retrieved from https://www.rebootwithjoe.com/how-mindfulness-can-impact-weight-loss/

Kubala, M. (2022, January 6). 16 Delicious High Protein Foods. Retrieved from https://www.healthline.com/nutrition/high-protein-foods

Longevity. (2020, May 20). Will A Detox Improve My Sex Life? Ask Dr Rascher. Retrieved from https://longevitylive.com/sex/detox-sex-life/

Longevity. (2022, June 7). 11 Ways a Detox will make You Feel Better. Retrieved from https://longevitywellnessworldwide.com/longevity-blog/11-ways-detox-will-make-you-feel-better/

Macey, D. (2019, April 12). Guide to Whole Grains. Retrieved from https://runningonrealfood.com/guide-to-whole-grains/

Mankermi, S. (2021, July 14). What I Eat in a Day: Malaika Arora reveals her diet secrets - Times of India. Retrieved from https://timesofindia.indiatimes.com/entertainment/hindi/bollywood/news/what-i-eat-in-a-day-malaika-arora-reveals-her-diet-secrets/articleshow/84405837.cms

Marketing The Conscious Club. (2019, May 23). Food & Chemicals. Retrieved from https://www.theconsciouschallenge.org/ecologicalfootprintbibleoverview/food-chemicals

Maser, R. (2018, January 26). 20 Health Benefits of Clean Eating. Retrieved from https://cleanfoodcrush.com/twenty-clean-eating-benefits/

Masterclass. (2021, May 28). How to Do Upward-Facing Dog: 3 Benefits of Upward Dog Pose. Retrieved from https://www.masterclass.com/articles/upward-facing-dog-guide#quiz-0

Mayle, W. (2021, June 11). One Incredible Side Effect of Dancing More Every Day, Says New Study. Retrieved from https://www.eatthis.com/news-side-effect-dancing/

Mayo Clinic. (2021a, March 12). Menopause weight gain: Stop the middle age spread. Retrieved from https://www.mayoclinic.org/healthy-lifestyle/womens-health/in-depth/menopause-weight-gain/art-20046058

Mayo Clinic. (2021b, April 20). Calf stretch. Retrieved from https://www.mayoclinic.org/diseases-conditions/muscle-cramp/multimedia/calf-stretch/img-20007902

Mayo Clinic. (2021c, May 17). Child's pose. Retrieved from https://www.mayoclinic.org/healthy-lifestyle/stress-management/multimedia/childs-pose/vid-20453580?reDate=17082022

Mayo Clinic. (2021d, June 17). Exercise intensity: How to measure it. Retrieved from https://www.mayoclinic.org/healthy-lifestyle/fitness/in-depth/exercise-intensity/art-20046887?reDate=17082022

Mayo Clinic. (2022). Stretching: Focus on flexibility. Retrieved from https://www.mayoclinic.org/healthy-lifestyle/fitness/in-depth/stretching/art-20047931?reDate=17082022

MedLine Plus. (n.d.). Aging changes in body shape. Retrieved from https://medlineplus.gov/ency/article/003998.htm

Menopause.org. (n.d.). Changes in Weight and Fat Distribution, Sexual Side Effects of Menopause | The North American Menopause Society, NAMS. Retrieved from https://www.menopause.org/for-women/sexual-health-menopause-online/changes-at-midlife/changes-in-weight-and-fat-distribution

mindbodygreen. (2019, January 19). How To Detox For Better Brain Health. Retrieved from https://www.mindbodygreen.com/articles/how-to-detox-for-better-brain-health

Mindful. (2021, November 23). What is Mindfulness? Retrieved from https://www.mindful.org/what-is-mindfulness/

Mullins, B. (2021, June 1). Grapefruit Smoothie. Retrieved from https://www.eatingbirdfood.com/grapefruit-detox-smoothie/

Munch Munch Yum. (2021, June 2). Best Detox Smoothies (+ 3-Day Cleanse Plan). Retrieved from https://munchmunchyum.com/detox-smoothie/

Ogle, M. (2021, May 31). Stretch Your Hip Flexors with Standing Lunges. Retrieved from https://www.verywellfit.com/hip-flexor-stretch-the-lunge-2704714

Osipov, O. (2022, August 12). 65 Quick and Easy Healthy Dinner Ideas.

Retrieved from https://ifoodreal.com/clean-eating-recipes-dinners/

Petre, A. (2019, September 5). What Is Refined Sugar? Retrieved from https://www.healthline.com/nutrition/refined-sugar

Physio Pedia. (n.d.). Single Knee to Chest Stretch. Retrieved from https://www.physio-pedia.com/Single_Knee_to_Chest_Stretch

Printablee. (n.d.). 10 Best Free Printable Weight Loss Logs - printablee.com. Retrieved from https://www.printablee.com/post_free-printable-weight-loss-logs_257926/

Pure Wow. (n.d.). Recipes | Easy Meal Ideas for Breakfast, Lunch, Dinner & Dessert. Retrieved from https://www.purewow.com/recipes

Radcliffe, S. (2019, January 18). Exercise Is Good for You, But Does It Really Affect Weight Loss? Retrieved from https://www.healthline.com/health-news/exercise-good-for-you-but-does-it-help-weight-loss#Exercise-doesnt-always-lead-to-weight-loss

Red Bull Editorial Team. (2022, January 21). Learn New Dance Moves at Home. Retrieved from https://www.redbull.com/in-en/how-to-learn-dance-at-home

Revord, J. (n.d.). Piriformis Muscle Stretch and Physical Therapy. Retrieved from https://www.spine-health.com/conditions/sciatica/piriformis-muscle-stretch-and-physical-therapy

Riopel, L. (2022, August 2). 28 Best Meditation Techniques for Beginners to Learn. Retrieved from https://positivepsychology.com/meditation-techniques-beginners/

Robinson, L. (2022, August 16). Organic Foods: What You Need to Know. Retrieved from https://www.helpguide.org/articles/healthy-eating/organic-foods.htm

School of Medicine and Public Health. (n.d.). Obesity by Age. Retrieved from https://www.wihealthatlas.org/obesity/age

Sears, B. (2021, March 19). 3 Exercises to Do (in Order) to Properly Progress Low Back Flexion. Retrieved from https://www.verywellhealth.com/low-back-flexion-exercise-p2-2696216

SkinnyMs. (2022, January 31). 21 Clean Lunches in Under 10 Minutes. Retrieved from https://skinnyms.com/21-clean-lunches-that-can-be-prepared-in-under-10-minutes/

Spritzler, F. (2019, January 17). 8 Health Benefits of Nuts. Retrieved from https://www.healthline.com/nutrition/8-benefits-of-nuts#

Stefanacci, R. (2022, August 4). Changes in the Body With Aging. Retrieved from https://www.msdmanuals.com

Stephens, B. (2022, August 3). How Mindfulness Helps You Lose Weight. Retrieved from https://www.aarp.org/health/healthy-living/info-2019/mindfulness-weight-loss.html

Stewart, G. (2019, May 28). Detox for Allergy Relief: The Detox-Allergy Connection. Retrieved from https://www.wraptique.com/blog/2019/5/28/detox-for-allergy-relief-the-detox-allergy-connection

Strube, A. (2022, June 16). How to Do Downward Dog for Inflexible Beginners. Retrieved from https://yogarove.com/how-to-do-downward-dog/

Tabackman, L., & Cassetty, S. (2021, April 23). The benefits of a sugar detox and 7 tips for how to do one effectively, according to dietitians. Retrieved from https://www.insider.com/guides/health/diet-nutrition/sugar-detox

The Gracious Pantry. (2019, May 18). 15 Clean Eating Lunches You Can Prep In 15 Minutes Or Less! Retrieved from https://www.thegraciouspantry.com/15-clean-eating-lunches-you-can-prep-in-15-minutes-or-less/

Thompson, J. (2021, October 1). What Tom Brady Eats in a Day. . . Retrieved from https://news.yahoo.com/tom-brady-eats-day-stay-183723483.html

Thorpe, M. (2020, October 27). 12 Science-Based Benefits of Meditation. Retrieved from https://www.healthline.com/nutrition/12-benefits-of-meditation

Tran, P. (2013, September 17). How to Do Easy Pose in Yoga. Retrieved from https://www.everydayyoga.com/blogs/guides/how-to-do-easy-pose-in-yoga

Tromans, C. (2019, April 26). This is what Gwyneth Paltrow eats in a day. Retrieved from https://www.beautycrew.com.au/gwyneth-paltrow-clean-eating-diet-plan

van Amburg, J. (2021, August 2). One Secret Exercise Trick That Women Over 50 Should Try Now. Retrieved from https://www.eatthis.com/news-dancing-exercise-menopause/

van de Walle, M. G. S. (2022, June 22). Full Body Detox: 9 Ways to Rejuvenate Your Body. Retrieved from https://www.healthline.com/nutrition/how-to-detox-your-body

Verywell Fit. (2021, July 16). Tackle Your First Yoga Balance Safely With Tree Pose. Retrieved from https://www.verywellfit.com/tree-pose-vrksasana-3567128

Walsh, G. (2021, February 15). 7 day detox plan to kick-start your metabolism and weight loss. Retrieved from https://www.goodto.com/wellbeing/7-day-detox-plan-59890

Winn, E. J. (2022, April 26). 50 Clean Eating Snacks. Retrieved from https://realsimplegood.com/50-clean-eating-snacks/

Zelman, K. (2010, January 28). The Truth About White Foods. Retrieved from https://www.webmd.com/diet/obesity/features/truth-about-white-foods

Printed in Great Britain
by Amazon

39665693R00126